I Know How You Feel

I Know How You Feel

THE JOY AND HEARTBREAK OF FRIENDSHIP IN WOMEN'S LIVES

F. Diane Barth

Houghton Mifflin Harcourt
Boston · New York
2018

For information about permission to reproduce selections
from this book, write to trade.permissions@hmhco.com or to
Permissions, Houghton Mifflin Harcourt Publishing Company,
3 Park Avenue, 19th Floor, New York, New York 10016.

hmhco.com

Library of Congress Cataloging-in-Publication Data is available.
ISBN 978-0-544-87027-7

Book design by Chrissy Kurpeski

Printed in the United States of America
DOC 10 9 8 7 6 5 4 3 2 1

The definitions of *betray, boundary,* and *empathy* are copyright
© 2016 by Houghton Mifflin Harcourt Publishing Company.
Adapted and reproduced by permission from *The American
Heritage Dictionary of the English Language, Fifth Edition.*

To Simon and Blair, with love,
as you begin your new life together

Contents

Introduction

When my son was going through the "terrible twos," he had a major temper tantrum on the sidewalk outside our apartment building. Unable to calm him, and knowing that the eyes of a number of my neighbors were on us, I became increasingly flustered. The building's doorman, whom my son adored, stepped in; kneeling down to my son at eye level, he quietly soothed him. After thanking the doorman profusely, I hurried upstairs with my now happy child.

Once in the apartment, I had no idea what to do next. Could a two-year-old understand that he had behaved badly? He was busily playing with his toys, but I was still rattled. I knew I needed to compose myself before I could figure out my next step. So I did what women have been doing since the telephone was invented. I called a friend.

When I had poured out the whole sad story, she chuckled quietly and said, "Poor you. I know just how you feel. It's so embarrassing not to be able to deal with your own kid." And then she told me about her own children's tantrums and some of the ways she had —and had not—dealt with them. By the time we had talked for ten minutes, I was calm and had decided to try to explain, in language a two-year-old could grasp, why his behavior was not okay.

Whether he understood anything I said in that conversation, I have no idea. But the incident has stayed with me, because it captures what women friends have been doing for one another throughout history: soothing, empathizing, advising, and understanding.

These are some of the wonderful benefits of our friendships with other women. We celebrate and mourn, talk and listen, and provide sustenance, companionship, and hope to one other. Women laugh and cry together, enhancing our good feelings and easing our bad ones.

But friendships between women do not always work so smoothly. I have been paying attention to, talking about, and working as a psychotherapist on women's friendships for years. In life and in my work I have seen many examples of these special relationships gone wrong. Hurt, anger, guilt, and sorrow are also part of women's friendships. And despite the widely held belief that women have deeply meaningful connections to one another, plenty of women simply do not find other women particularly supportive or interesting, and never have understood what all of the "friendship fuss," as one of my clients puts it, is about. Women are supposed to be good at friendships. At least that's what we hear and see all the time — not only in the media, but in serious psychological literature as well. But the truth, as Luise Eichenbaum and Susie Orbach[1] write in their book *Between Women,* is that we have put women's friendships on a pedestal, idealizing some aspects of these relationships while ignoring others. When it comes to close bonds with other women, many of us feel insecure and anxious.

I hear about these anxieties daily. For instance, one woman told me, "I just found out that my friend is getting promoted. I should be happy for her, but I'm not. What's the matter with me? What kind of friend am I?"

Another, working on a toast for a friend's wedding, said, "I'm so worried that I'm not going to say the right things. We have a complicated relationship. I mean, I love her to death, but we've had our moments too. I want to say some funny things, but I don't want any of it to sound mean. Oh, why did I ever let her talk me into doing this?"

A young mother told me that she had been neglecting her friends since the birth of her second child. "I miss them. They probably hate me by now. I never have time to talk. I don't know what any of them are doing."

A recent divorcée asked, "What is it with my friends? Do they think I don't need them anymore now that I'm on my own? Where did they all go?"

What do we do when a friend deserts or betrays us? What happens when a close friend is doing something we don't like or don't approve of? Does a good friend keep her mouth closed or give unwanted advice? What *is* a good friend, anyway?

In my search for answers, I interviewed many women, from all over the world, and with a wide range of backgrounds, personalities, and lifestyles. Some of them were gifted at friendship, others had always felt awkward about these relationships, and some told me that they had become more skilled and comfortable as they got older. Many had never given the subject of women's friendships much thought, although as soon as I brought it up, they said, "Oh, that's so important!" Others often worried about many of the same things that concerned my clients. But whether they questioned their own friendship abilities — and even their self-worth — as well as the depth and quality of their bonds, few had ever spoken about these matters to anyone else, often struggling silently with the complex and sometimes painful sides of these all-important relationships, and wondering what they could do to make things better next time.

In writing *I Know How You Feel,* I wanted to find out what women thought about questions like these: Why do we feel so unprotected when it comes to women friends? Does the discomfort go away with age and experience? Or does it intensify? Why does a contact from the past fill us with such powerful and confusing feelings? And, of course, what makes women's friendships so fulfilling that some of us stay connected for a lifetime, and others say they couldn't live without their women friends?

Many of the women I met blamed themselves for the problems in their friendships. They thought they had done something wrong, had somehow failed at friendship. A working mother in her thirties said something that I heard often, albeit in a variety of forms. "I look at all of the Facebook posts by women I know, and then I compare my group of 'friends' to theirs. I'm embarrassed to even tell you how many. But it's a measly little number. What's wrong with me? Why don't I have more friends?" Shame, embarrassment, fear of being criticized or hurt — all of these feelings keep women quiet about their ability to make and keep friendships.

As a psychotherapist I have learned that the first step toward change often comes when we put into words what may never have been spoken or even thought before. In *I Know How You Feel* I integrate theory and research with stories from real women, giving you an opportunity to think about, understand, and perhaps talk about your own secret fears and doubts about your friendships and the roles they do — and don't — play in your life.

Both everyday experience and research data show that attachments to other women are important to our mental health. Without these important connections, we often feel lonely, unprotected, *and* self-critical. Yet despite the popular image of mutual support and feminine bonding, friendships can also *create* difficulties. We may not say it out loud, but many of us also feel exposed and anxious in the company of our women friends. Convinced that we were absent the day that everyone else was taught to negotiate such alliances, we feel bad about ourselves, which of course means we are less likely to talk to anyone about our so-called inadequacies; and this means we feel ever more alone and inadequate.

I Know How You Feel is all about other women who feel the same way you do — women whose friendships bring them love and pain, solace and frustration, heartbreak and joy.

Magical, meaningful, and surprisingly difficult, these connections are filled with contradictions. They can make us feel simultaneously special and outcast, loved and unlovable, vulnerable and strong, helpful and useless, angry and happy, alone and lonely, supportive and held. Developmental theory, recent research on women's relationships, and real women who tell their stories will help you understand more about your own friendships. With new clarity and understanding, you may find yourself making changes in your idea of what a friend is, your interactions with friends, and the way you want to be and have a friend. You might not even notice some of the shifts you make. But, as any psychotherapist will tell you, small changes can make a big difference in how you feel.

I Know How You Feel

1

⁓

How Should a Friendship Begin?

UZANNE, A WORKING MOTHER WITH ONE CHILD and a second on the way, came to therapy because she was feeling more alone than ever before. "I should be so happy," she said. "I have everything I've ever wanted. A job I love, a great husband, a terrific kid . . ." She looked up with a grin. "Well, at least they're great and terrific most of the time. But I feel like something's missing.

"It seems that when you go through different times in your life, you change," she said. "It's not just that you don't have time even to pee, let alone see your friends. Your focus is different. You're different. Some friends can handle the differences, but some can't. It's painful when the other person didn't sign up for who you have become. And it's scary to try to reach out to new people. I mean, the women I know don't have any more time than I do. They don't need a new friend . . ."

When I began writing about women's friendships, I was amazed at how many people wanted to talk to me about their own experiences, in and out of therapy. Almost everyone had a story to share and questions about how other women managed these important connections. The stories frequently had to do with beginning a friendship. Women of all ages talked about having fewer friends than they did when they were younger.

Suzanne's words echoed in my mind as, over and over again, I heard, "I used to make friends so easily, but as I've gotten older it has gotten harder. Why is it tougher now than it was when I was young?" Many women wondered if they were the only ones who struggled with this difficulty. Like Suzanne, they believed that other women were not looking for new friends. As one vibrant single woman in her forties put it, "Rejection hurts, no matter how nicely or gently it's done."

Recent graduates talked about how much they missed their college buddies and how much harder it was to find friends away from campus life. New mothers like Suzanne spoke of the difficulty of finding new friends in the early stages of motherhood, and single women told me about their struggles to find friends who shared their interests. Like these women, whether you are in your twenties or your eighties or anywhere in between, whether you have always been part of a close-knit group or have had one or two close friends at a time, you may suddenly realize that you are having trouble beginning new friendships. If so, you are not alone.

Research shows a peak in the number of friends during our early twenties, followed by a steady decline as we move into our late twenties.[1] A twenty-six-year-old dental hygienist put it this way: "I barely get to see my old friends these days. Some of us are in serious relationships and others are busy looking for one. Our jobs take up huge amounts of time. I have friends at work, but we don't get together socially. There's just not the easy kind of connecting anymore." Her experience is not at all uncommon. Making new friends gets even more difficult for many of us as we move through the next stages of life. According to an article in the *New York Times*, "As people approach midlife, the days of youthful exploration, when life felt like one big blind date, are fading. Schedules compress, priorities change, and people often become pickier in what they want in their friends."[2]

I learned long ago from my psychotherapy clients that some women make friends easily, almost without effort, while others find it hard. I also found that these patterns sometimes vary over time. Starting a new job, a relationship, or a family can be challenging to established friendships and may demand new ways of connecting. A move, a divorce, a job loss, or the illness or death of loved ones can force us to start over. One study[3] found that the mythical seven-year itch sometimes exists in friendships as well as other relationships. Some friendships do last, of course, but many are purposely altered over time, some end abruptly and sometimes painfully, and others simply get lost in the passage of years. We change physically, emotionally, and intellectually. Our social situation alters. Elena, the narrator of Elena Ferrante's powerful fictional saga about women's friendship, describes some of the difficulty of maintaining and restoring old, important relationships. She says, "To regain our old intimacy we would have had to speak our secret thoughts, but I didn't have the strength to find the words and she, who perhaps had the strength, didn't have the desire."[4]

How do we make new friends when we need and want them?

Only Connect

I started posing the question "How do women connect?" to every woman who would talk with me, which turned out to be almost anyone with whom I came into contact. Clients, friends, colleagues, and relatives shared stories about how they found new women friends. I discussed the subject with students, supervisees, strangers, and followers of my *Psychology Today* blog. Mounds of evidence showed that there was no "one size fits all" formula for how women connect to one another. Some women said they sometimes found new friends simply by talking to other people. Others said that friends found them. Quite a few described themselves as "shy" or "introverted" and said that they needed someone else, a partner, a spouse, another friend, a colleague, or even a child to help them make new connections.

According to popular belief, women get together to talk about feelings, while men get together to do something. Yet many of the women who responded to my questions told me that they made connections through activities: taking a class, walking in the neighborhood, or attending church, temple, or mosque. One recent college grad captured the experience of many who were looking to replace the easy camaraderie of campus friendships. She said, "Things like intramural sports and online meet-up groups are huge among my friends. I started volunteering at a food co-op to meet more people who love food like I do."

Some of the older women who talked to me were less comfortable about the fact that some of their more recent friendships had developed from activities. A working mother said, "Girlfriends are supposed to be the people you open your heart to, not the people you see at work or your goodhearted neighbor — all you have in common with her is your kids and the neighborhood where you live. But I don't have time to talk to, let alone see, anybody else these days."

A fifty-five-year-old woman who joined a memoir-writing group when her youngest child left for college said, "I love this group. We talk about what we're writing or not writing about, about how hard the writing process is, and about books we've read that we think other people in the group will enjoy or find useful. Sometimes we talk about our children or our partners. We also talk about our lives, because we're writing our histories. But we hardly ever talk about feelings." She too sometimes worried that this lack of heart-to-heart conversation meant that there was something missing. "It doesn't seem like these could be real friendships," she said. "It's the way I think of guys connecting—around sports or something. Maybe I think it's just not very feminine, or I guess womanly, to get together with your women friends to *do* something."

While many women newly graduated from college freely acknowledge that, as one young professional put it, "There are some things that aren't as fun unless you're doing it with somebody else," many older women worry that there is something wrong with needing friends to share activities. A radiologist in her late forties said, "I was brought up to be independent. I should be able to do anything I want by myself. So I'm kind of embarrassed when I want a buddy to go out with me." But she and many other women of all ages agreed that it was just more fun to do things with someone else, even if that person was not a close friend.

Many shared a belief that women's friendships should begin with some kind of magnetic attraction or spontaneous bonding that few had experienced since their late teens. An amazing number of women described these relationships — the kinds that usually start sometime in adolescence. Liz, a petite, dark-haired woman with a contagious smile, works in management at a large retail chain in a small town in the southwestern United States. "I wouldn't live anywhere else," she said. "But when my family moved here when I was twelve, I thought I was going to die." Liz is Chinese American. Her parents, who had come to the United States as young adults, moved with their two children to the Southwest because of her father's work. "There were practically no other Chinese and few Asians of any sort. In my old school, I had a mix of friends, Asian and non-Asian. In my new school, I kept getting put together with a Vietnamese kid who barely spoke English. I was so miserable." But then, one day as she walked through the cafeteria looking for a place to eat, she saw Eileen.

"Something about her seemed so right . . . I didn't have the words for it at the time, but I just knew we were soulmates. She'll tell you the same thing. She saw me walking toward her table in the cafeteria, made eye contact, and just scooched over, patting the bench next to her. For the rest of high school, we sat together at lunch. Other girls came and went from our table, but from that day on, Eileen and I were a pair."

Movies, television programs, novels, and social media reinforce these images of the perfect match, occurring most often in high school or college, as the way that women's friendships should begin. Images of the pop singer Taylor Swift and her twinning squad-goal friend Karlie Kloss stir fantasies of bosom girlfriends. Perhaps pop culture simply emphasizes what several studies[5] have shown: we seek out friends who are like us. In our hearts, we would like to have something like these squads who move in the same social and professional world *and* go out of their way to look, sound, and be like one another.

Of course, we do not all believe in these images. As one twenty-something put it, "The whole celebrity social media BFF [best friend forever] situation is so strange. You have to wonder sometimes if they are actually friends. And then, why does everyone care so much?" Popular culture offers other ways of thinking about women's friendships too. *Orange Is the New Black* is only one of a number of contemporary TV shows with far more nuanced images of female friendships.[6] Still, there is an emotional and psychological pull toward the soulmate version of friendship.

In his classic Narnia series, C. S. Lewis describes this kind of perfect-match moment between Lucy, a human girl, and a fantasy sea person whom she glimpses briefly: "The girl looked up [from under the ocean] and stared straight into Lucy's face. Neither could speak to the other and in a moment the Sea Girl dropped astern. But . . . Lucy had liked that girl and she felt certain the girl had liked her. In that one moment they had somehow become friends. There does not seem to be much chance of their meeting again in that world or any other. But if ever they do they will rush together with their hands held out."[7]

These instant connections seem magical, yet they are the result of many complicated factors, including individual personalities and life experiences. They also almost always happen in relation to a very specific stage of life. Liz and Eileen's friendship changed over time, as any relationship must. But their early, special connection became the template of friendship for the future. Whether they had once been in such a relationship or had only read about or seen them unfold for others, many of the women I spoke with longed for just that kind of spontaneous link with another woman.

A Perfect Match, and Then . . .

A "perfect match" is one way, albeit not the only way, that we can discover more about ourselves and others. What looks and feels like a magical connection requires a kind of trust and openness that exists when we are young and often disappears as we get older. It also demands a somewhat malleable sense of self, that is, openness to different views of who you are. This ability to be flexible about our very identity diminishes as we get older.

Liz was especially animated as she continued her story about that first encounter with Eileen.

"We didn't want to stop talking, ever. We didn't want to go back to class, and if we hadn't been such 'good girls,' we would have just skipped out and played hooky for the rest of the day. When school was over, we didn't want to head back to our own homes, either. We spent hours on the phone that night. Neither one of us wanted to hang up, even with our moms yelling at us to get off for dinner and homework. We did finally stop talking long enough to eat, but we got back on the phone and just stayed on the line, not talking, but keeping each other company while we both did our assignments. And we kept it up for the whole time we were in high school."

The stage of life in which we begin to develop close attachments to peers outside our family is when we start to become the person we will be. For Liz and Eileen, as for many adolescents, what looked like magic was a relationship that gave them each a sense of identity and security during a time so often characterized by confusion, self-doubt, and a sense of not-knowing. "I'm like Eileen," Liz could tell herself. Since she admired everything about her friend, she could feel good about herself as well. Still, from the outside, this relationship looked like anything but a path toward individual and separate identities.

"We felt like we were sisters, separated at birth. Twins with different physical appearances." Liz was short and delicately built, with straight dark hair, and Eileen was tall with a full figure and wild, light brown curls. "We were outsiders in the world of blond Southern girls. Even though we didn't look like each other, either, we shared the same feelings underneath."

They also shared a sense of being different from their own families. While Liz's parents had emigrated from China, Eileen's were first-generation American Jews from Europe. Both families wanted their children to remain true to their family's heritage while also finding a way to assimilate, a complicated yet common expectation for many children of recent immigrants.

The fact that they spent all of their time together and did everything as a duo disturbed both girls' parents. "They didn't want to end our closeness, but they worried that we were bad for each other, that we would destroy our individuality in order to protect our friendship."

Although Liz added after a moment, "Well, they were right too, of course. Eventually that need to be similar was our downfall."

"Twinning" is a popular term that shows up on social media and the Internet. It refers to friends who have similar thoughts, tastes, and interests. It is also a psychological term that captures a significant aspect of the beginning of a friendship, and not just in adolescence. For psychotherapists, "twinship" is a step on the developmental path toward mature relationships and self-knowledge.[8] When you find someone who shares your thoughts, feelings, and attitudes, it reinforces your sense that you are all right, that what you believe and who you believe yourself to be are both fine, even normal.

Twinning adolescents might share everything from clothes and music to secrets and crushes. When we feel that we have found a twin, we also have found a way of knowing ourselves better. A twin not only shows us what we might look like, but she also validates our feelings by having the same emotions herself. Of course, when one member of the dyad refuses to accept any differences, a twinship can be destructive. This demand for sameness can destroy the quest for personal identity that is a healthy aspect of these relationships.

The need to know that our feelings make sense to another person stays with us long after adolescence. Contemporary attachment theory tells us that the desire for connection is a basic human need. This longing is part of our makeup and lasts from birth to death, just like the need for food to eat and oxygen to breathe, says John Bowlby,[9] the British psychologist who brought these ideas to the attention of the psychoanalytic world.

Twinning can look and feel similar to romantic and even sexual love. The couples-therapy guru Harville Hendrix's description of love at first sight sounds a lot like friendship at first sight. He writes, "Your eyes meet (perhaps across a crowded room). Heart palpitations start." And the fairy tale begins. Shared meals, shared laughter, and "hours looking forward to your next time together. Maybe you'll see a movie or simply hang out — talking about everything and nothing."[10]

For the most part, twinning is neither sexual nor romantic, although it can sometimes include sexual experimentation. While these bonds are often not permanent, they can be a kind of training for more mature, intimate relationships.

Twinning does not work as well as we get older, however. You may still have moments when you feel, maybe with a mix of surprise and pleasure, that someone gets you simply because she is so much like you. It is normal and even healthy to look for new friends who are similar to you,[11] but as we mature we also look for friends who are different in some ways. We grow to understand that we get a great deal from friends who bring their own personalities and interests to the table.

Self-Protection

If you missed out on the twinning experience in adolescence, you are definitely not alone. As I gathered information on women's friendships, I frequently heard, "I'm not like other women; I don't make friends easily" or "I don't have lots of women friends." Some told me they were closer to their boyfriend or husband than to women. Many shared that they did not like talking about "girl stuff" like "clothes, exercise, weight, hairstyles, children, food, men, decorating, or gossip." Yet not one of these qualities makes you either a "bad" friend or different from many other women.

I began to notice a fear of rejection running through most of these "I'm not like other women" stories. Women talked about fears of being hurt or vulnerable when they made the first tentative steps toward a new relationship with another woman. Even some who said they made friends easily often felt a twinge of anxiety before embarking upon a new connection.

These concerns often originate in the experience of adolescent friendships. Many of us carry memories of one or more of these relationships ending painfully, leaving us feeling bruised and tender.

This is what happened to Liz when Eileen abandoned her to join a group of other girls. Suddenly they were no longer best friends. Eileen simply told Liz she was too busy to hang out anymore. Badly hurt, Liz withdrew from what had been the most important part of her life. "I put all of my energy into my schoolwork and my college applications," she said. "I told myself that I would find a new friend when I got to university." Yet for some years after their "breakup," Liz found herself worrying that any new friendships would end badly as well. "I stopped trusting other women," she told me. "And I didn't trust myself, either. I had clearly missed some signals that things had shifted with Eileen. I didn't know if I would see them this time around."

If you have ever been through a version of this kind of breakup, like Liz you may go on to doubt your own perceptions and question the validity of any good feelings you have about a new acquaintance.

"She was my soulmate, and she betrayed me," Liz said. "How could I ever trust anyone again?"

Not surprisingly, Eileen's side of the story was different. She was frightened about what would happen when they graduated. Liz was focused on getting into a top-tier college. "I wasn't as good a student as you," she told Liz. "And my family wouldn't have let me go away to college, no matter how well I did. I was hurt and angry. You didn't seem to have any idea about how I was feeling. And I was ashamed that I didn't want to support you. I wanted you to go to the state university with me."

At the time, she could not explain any of these feelings to Liz or even fully put them into words to herself. She knew only that she felt relieved and pleased when a group of girls wanted to be friends with her. "I didn't feel like I was abandoning you, because I felt as though you had already left me behind. It didn't occur to me that you would be so hurt."

The truth is that even healthy twinships inevitably lead to disappointment. At some point or another, twinning friends have to begin to separate in order to continue the psychological work of developing individual identities. "Optimal disappointment,"[12] in which the letdown is small enough to be managed either within the relationship or by turning to other supports, such as friends and family, helps us manage the loss and grow as people. When this happens, we develop better friendship skills.

But when the pain is too great, we end up trying to protect ourselves from future hurt. That's often when we find ourselves distrusting others or doubting our instincts about them.

Previous disappointment and current feelings of vulnerability can make it hard to start a new friendship. When you are drawn to another woman, you may think of all the reasons there are for being careful. You do not want to get hurt again, so you may sometimes avoid her. You might be slow to return her phone calls or texts.

Or maybe you are feeling vulnerable because of something that is going on in your life. Perhaps you have been ill recently, or someone you love is not doing well. You might be overwhelmed by responsibility or having a hard time in your marriage or at work. Maybe you feel like a failure because you have never had children, or the children you have are not doing well. Maybe you are convinced you are too old to start again.

A degree of self-protection is both normal and healthy. Yet sometimes the defenses we build to protect ourselves interfere with our ability to have a rich and meaningful life. Sometimes just when you are most afraid of making a new friend is the best time to find one. The need to balance taking care of yourself with taking appropriate risks is part of what Brené Brown[13] terms "daring greatly."

Many potential friends will understand that in a busy, over-scheduled life, going for a quick run or taking a yoga class together sometimes makes more sense than meeting for a long chat over a meal. But if you continue to keep a new friend at a distance, if you never find time for even a quick visit, you might reassess your interest in her. Or the problem might not be with other women, but with your own worries about getting close. If you are, for instance, always going to the gym or staying late at work instead of getting together with a woman you think could become a friend, it's possible you are protecting yourself from some danger that you have not spelled out for yourself. A new friendship might be a painful reminder of a lost friend. A new friend might not reflect back the "you" that you want to be. You could be afraid of being overwhelmed by a new friend's needs or, on the other hand, of not getting your own needs met. Perhaps you are worried about being rejected.

What You Can Do

As adults, we seldom become best buddies instantly the way Liz and Eileen did. This is partly because we know about the possible downside and even the danger of these connections. It is also partly because we are often just too busy to give up all of our time and energy to one person, the way best friends can do when they are young. Yet almost every woman and most of the men with whom I spoke longed for the special connection that they believed to be part of women's friendships.

Holding on to the image of a perfect match can make it difficult to find and develop new friendships as you get older. If you are in the market for some new female companionship, it can help to remind yourself that friendships come in many shapes and styles. You might start by looking at some of the less-than-perfect connections that already exist in your life. A casual friend with whom you occasionally have coffee can be invaluable at times. A coworker who has children the same age as yours may not have any more time available than you do. As a colleague, she is probably not the right person with whom to share all of your self-doubts and insecurities, but she might be a source of sympathy and support when you are trying to figure out how to get your son started on his homework while you try to meet a deadline.

If you tend to be a little shy, try to find someone else to introduce you to other women. One professional woman in her late thirties told me that several of her closest friendships had developed only after a mutual acquaintance made the initial contact for her. A soft-spoken widow said that her social life had revolved around her outgoing husband. After his death a woman she knew only slightly had invited her to join a book club, and although she had been a little reluctant to join at first, she eventually did go. While she did not become best friends with any of the women, some became supportive and interesting companions for a variety of activities.

Even if you prefer one-on-one connections, joining a group can be a way to make new contacts. A group can be formally organized around an activity like writing or reading or attending the theater, or it can occur spontaneously as you and a neighbor walk your dogs. Research[14] shows that participating in some activity, even if you do not particularly enjoy it, is one of the best ways to meet and make new friends. For instance, an active sixty-two-year-old who had moved to a new home told me that she did not usually go looking for friends. "They find me," she said. "But this neighborhood is so quiet that I wasn't running into anyone. I finally met one person who told me about a group of neighbors who were part of a regular walking group. I hate walking, but I decided to join it anyway, just to meet some of them. I had to push myself to go the first time, but my reward was that I met someone who started complaining about how much she hated to exercise. It turned out that we didn't have a whole lot of other things in common, but I had found a buddy!"

If you are having difficulties finding a group activity, you might try some of the ever-growing and very popular apps that aim to fill exactly that need. In an article on BuzzFeed, Chelsea Pippin has listed and described seventeen of these apps, including ones where you can locate folks with interests similar to your own, from dog owners to world travelers to cheese lovers.[15]

But how do you take the first steps toward a new friendship while also protecting yourself? One way is to proceed slowly and even with caution. When going to a new meet-up for an activity, it can be good to go with another woman, even a casual acquaintance. Who knows, she might turn out to be a new activity buddy!

There is also nothing wrong with allowing space between contacts with a friend, new or old, as you get older. Unlike the almost merged quality of friendship that can exist when we are young, adult contact often has to take into account the separate and busy lives of both women.

Working around both of your schedules may mean that you see one another only once in a great while. It can help, if it feels appropriate, to tell a new acquaintance that you would like to get to know her better, but that you do not have a lot of disposable time. If you are not comfortable spelling this out, or you worry that she might feel you are pushing her away, find other, more subtle ways to communicate that you would like to see her as soon as you get a minute to breathe. It can help simply to set a time, even if it is weeks away.

Beginning new friendships *is* different as we get older, although you may not have stopped to think about these changes before now. Or, if you have noticed, you might, like other women, have blamed yourself for your inadequacies as a friend. But as we have seen, these changes in how we make friends are simply part of life. We learn that women need and want close friendships — all of the time or some of the time. But what is it, exactly, that we want? To begin to answer this question, it will help to look more closely at our definition of women's friendships.

2

~

What Are Women's Friendships?

ONE NIGHT WHEN MY HUSBAND AND I WERE HAVing dinner with several other couples, I mentioned that I was writing a book on women's friendships. Kevin, a colleague and friend, said, "I've always wished that I could have friendships like you women do." Touched by his words and by the longing in his voice, I asked if he could say what he believed was special about women's friendships. He said, "The ability to talk about your deepest feelings and thoughts with each other. I think that must give you a sense of being deeply connected in a way that we men don't get from each other."

Around the table I saw many different reactions. Two men and one of the women were nodding in agreement. But one woman shook her head and said, "That's a romantic fantasy. I don't have friends like that. I don't think many women really do." Another woman remarked, "Oh, I do. I don't know how I would get through life without my close women friends." Someone else said that she saw many of her friends only occasionally, but that when they got together they couldn't stop talking. "And it's not all about deep feelings. We just love to share what's going on in our lives."

A man said, "I don't know. I've seen a lot of awful stuff go on between women who are supposed to be friends." But then Kevin answered, "Yes, that's true, I've seen that too. But still, there's some kind of emotional connection that we men don't get to."

How to Define Women's Friendships

As was clear at the dinner table that night, it is not easy to find a single, universally agreed upon definition of women's friendships. In her book *Connecting: The Enduring Power of Female Friendship,* the journalist Sandy Sheehy tells us that this is because friendship is "what philosophers call a fuzzy concept," without specific social or legal rules that everyone agrees on.[1] Geoffrey Greif, a psychologist who studies these special relationships, writes that there is "a great variation that exists in individual definitions of and experiences with friendships," yet in his research he found that certain phrases, such as "being understood, trusting, being able to depend on somebody, doing things together, and finding commonalities," are often used to describe these bonds.[2]

A Harris interactive poll of over six hundred women between the ages of twenty-five and fifty-five across the United States also found that "support" was a key word used to describe friendships between women, although the form of support was varied. For example, 81 percent said that support involved friends allowing them to vent, 76 percent described laughing as crucial, 69 percent said their friends cheered them up, 68 percent said that simply being able to talk to another adult was important, and 66 percent said friends supported them by offering advice.[3]

The women I spoke with also used words like "warmth," "understanding," "connection," "trust," and "empathy" to talk about friendship. One thirty-eight-year-old described a woman she called a "model friend. She is interested in your interests, but doesn't have any difficulty asking for the same from you. There's reciprocity in the friendship. She can be on-the-surface or more profound. She is very responsive and respectful of others. She also has good boundaries, good self-esteem, and self-confidence."

Many women told me that they made friends in their communities, their religious groups, their jobs, and other places where they found people who were similar to them, which meshed with research findings that we often choose friends whose values and lifestyles are the same as our own.[4] Researchers have found the same thing I heard repeatedly from women all over the world: many women define a friend as "someone you can be yourself with," "someone you trust," and "someone you can call on for help."[5]

But others told me that they enjoyed friends who could offer them a different perspective from their own. Some women said that being able to talk about things they couldn't tell their spouse or partner was part of their definition of friendship. Yet others said that their partners or spouses were their closest friends.

The truth is that how you define the word "friendship" depends on a variety of factors, including your age, life stage, individual personality, background, history, and previous experiences. A casual acquaintance who smiles when you pass on the street, a friendly colleague you see only at the office, or a former college roommate who shares your deepest secrets — you might call all of them your friends.

In the end, as the philosopher Alexander Nehamas says, all

friendships, despite being "consistently praised as one of life's greatest gifts,"[6] are intensely complex and nuanced. And as the narrator of the novel *Enchanted Islands*[7] puts it, "Friendships between women are complicated."

Yet while I found that friendship has different meanings for different women, I also discovered some common threads running through women's descriptions of what they expected from and gave to their friendships. Let's take a look at some of these common denominators.

An Emotional Connection

While a desire to connect to others is part of human nature, there is a general belief that women may be both hard-wired and socially encouraged to be more in tune with emotions than men are.[8] So it would seem natural that many definitions of friendship include emotional connection. Daniel Goleman, who coined the term "emotional intelligence," says that women are more "emotionally empathic" than men.[9] Studies have found that our brains respond to other people's feelings as though *we are feeling the emotions ourselves.*[10] And as the author Deborah Tannen illustrates, "we stay with the feelings, whereas men's brains tend to go quickly toward finding solutions."[11] Of course, this is not an all-or-nothing equation. Not every woman is equally empathic, and many of us are terrific problem-solvers. And certainly many men have a great capacity for emotional empathy. But the capacity to *understand,* often without words, is one of the defining characteristics of women's friendships.

One woman in her forties echoed the words of many when she described a good friend who, she said, "is a person who intuitively knows how to find and create friendships. She is warm and engaged, and you always know she's interested in what you have to say. She connects emotionally with you, but she isn't intrusive. She's just with you, wherever you're at."

We tend to pull friends from social categories that are somewhat similar to our own, probably[12] because such similarities can give us a jump-start on shared emotional experiences and mutual understanding. One businesswoman told me that she had two best friends. One, she said, was a lesbian from a Polish American background. The other was African American. "We get each other in part because we are all marginalized. But Jayla and I bonded as two smart, successful Black women. We know it's a hard position to be in, and we push each other to make our voices heard in places where we are being ignored, like in a business meeting where people think we're just there because of affirmative action."

A good friend sympathizes when you're down and celebrates when you're happy. She resonates with your feelings, and expects you to do the same with her. In fact, as we all know, to have a friend, you have to be a friend. But it's easy to be empathic with someone when she is feeling just what you are feeling, or just what you might feel in the same situation. Sometimes we have to stretch ourselves to understand — or to let someone in enough for her to understand us.

Someone Who Gets You

Whether talking about a friend they have known for years or one they were just connecting with, women frequently say that one of the defining characteristics of their relationship is that they "just get each other."

What exactly does this mean? Reciprocity, or a sense of mutuality, seemed to be important in almost every definition that I heard. Feeling understood, known, and appreciated, *and* understanding, knowing, and appreciating a friend were at the core of almost all of the successful friendships I heard about.

Psychoanalysts believe that we all need others who can affirm our sense of who we are, who can know us as we know ourselves.[13] The British psychoanalyst D. W. Winnicott called the experience of being seen as you really are "a sacred moment," because he believed that it was such an important part of healthy emotional life.[14]

But we women are good at looking for commonalities even in situations where it would seem there are none.

Richelle, a nurse in her forties, told me that she and her husband had moved into a family-friendly neighborhood when they started trying to get pregnant. Two and a half years later they still had no children, while numerous friends and relatives, including both Richelle's sister and her sister-in-law, had conceived and had babies. While out for a jog one Saturday morning, Richelle noticed that a new couple had moved into a house down the block. A woman of about Richelle's age came out of the house, a baby in a snuggly on her chest. Normally a friendly person, Richelle could not bring herself to stop to introduce herself or welcome the other woman to the neighborhood. She simply nodded in greeting as she jogged by.

"I didn't want to talk to her," Richelle said. "I already had too many friends and family with babies, and as happy as I was for them, I was sad and angry for myself. It was hard enough hiding those feelings from everyone I already knew. I couldn't be all nice and gaga over one more infant."

One day at the grocery store Richelle ran into the neighbor, Adeli, in the vegetable aisle. "She asked me how I liked the neighborhood, and her eyes were so warm and understanding that I felt really comfortable chatting with her. At that point I did ask about her baby — whether it was a girl or a boy, what her name was, and how old she was. She asked me if I had children, and somehow I was telling her what was going on, and crying, and she was rubbing my back. We left the grocery store and she invited me to her house, and we talked for hours. Even though she wasn't in the same spot as me, she just got my pain in a way no one else seemed to."

The ability to read another person's nonverbal emotional cues is called "cognitive empathy" and appears, according to some research, to be significantly stronger in women than in men.[15] It seems to be a key component of the sense of being understood that goes into many women's friendships. And it is central to the image that my friend Kevin was describing that night at dinner. There are questions about whether this is a trait we are born with or one that we are trained by our cultures to develop, but in either case, women tend to show a greater tendency to read and respond to the emotional aspect of nonverbal cues than do men.

Emotional and cognitive empathy is an important tool in parenting infants who have no words with which to explain what they are feeling. The wish for an understanding friend who is attuned to that unverbalized part of ourself is closely related to those early needs. When a friend's face and tone of voice reflect that she knows in her own body what we are feeling, we do not simply feel deeply understood. One of my clients said it most clearly, although many women told me something similar: we feel held in these moments, with an almost physical feeling of safety and well-being.

Empathy is complicated, however. It can also involve knowing that a friend needs space or silence. Sometimes it means *not* offering sympathy. There are times when even the most well-intentioned kind words or sympathetic expression can feel intrusive, pitying, or even condescending. An empathic friend may intuitively know that even a hug could be too much at such moments.

Mutual Respect

Women told me that they needed to respect their friends, and needed to know that their friends respected them. They might not admire or respect everything about a good friend, but without the sense that, as one thirty-one-year-old put it, "there are things I really appreciate and value about her, and I know she feels the same way about me," a friendship is not likely to survive for long. "I need to know that she's a good person," said a woman in her forties. "And I let her know what I like and admire about her."

This mutual respect often means comprehending what a friend needs and doesn't need from you. To be a friend you may need to respect a friend's boundaries, even if you momentarily feel left out or rejected by her. Understanding also means not taking her behavior personally. A forty-eight-year-old hairstylist told me that her best friend had periods of withdrawing from the world. "I've come to understand that it's not personal when she doesn't get back to me for days at a time," she said. "It's not about *me*. It's just that she's down and she needs her space. But a long time ago I also figured out that she didn't want radio silence from me during those times. I didn't think too much about it, but I sent her a text saying just 'Thinking about you. Love ya.'

"When she felt better, she told me she was so grateful that I didn't push or intrude, but that I let her know I was there for her. I think it was important to her to know that she hadn't disappeared from my thoughts, even though she had disappeared from my daily life. And I couldn't have done that if I took her withdrawal to mean she didn't care about me anymore."

Letting Stuff Slide

Mutual respect can go only so far. Liking is crucial to any friendship. One study found that a kind of "interpersonal chemistry" draws us together in the first place and helps us get through rough spots.[16] Two thirty-six-year-old longtime friends told me, "We didn't like each other at first. But some kind of energy between us kept pulling us together. And after a while, we realized that we really do like each other. We're very different, so we still run into moments where we don't like each other. But by now we know that there's so much that we do like that we can let the other stuff slide." They also talked about the importance of sharing their positive feelings. "You don't always remember to tell a friend how much you appreciate her. We try not to take each other for granted," said one, while the other nodded agreement.

Acknowledging the positive makes it easier to tolerate one another's flaws — at least to a certain extent. One forty-two-year-old told me, "I have a friend I love, but I can't eat a meal with her. She makes so much noise when she eats that I can't digest my own food. I've even told her, and asked her to try to eat more quietly when I'm around, but she doesn't believe that she really makes noise. Because she's important to me, I do eat with her, but we also do a lot of other things together. I think a lot of friendship is about compromise. That's what makes it work."

In Times of Trouble

Many of the women I spoke with defined a friend as someone who had their back. They could turn to those friends in times of trouble. But occasionally the person you think you can count on is not the one who comes through. And perhaps even more surprisingly, the person who turns out to be a really good friend was not even on your radar before you needed her.

That's how it was for Alysha when she was diagnosed with Lyme disease in her late twenties. "It sidelined me," said this tiny woman, who is now a ball of energy. "The first symptom was total fatigue, which wasn't like me at all. I've always had enough energy to fuel four or five people." After a series of misdiagnoses, during which she was told that she was suffering from depression, chronic fatigue syndrome, or leukemia, her doctors discovered and began treating the correct disease. "The treatment didn't work for a while," she said. "If I was tired before, I was completely nonfunctional during the first part of the treatment." Her joints hurt terribly and there was a question of damage to her nerves and her heart.

Her friends were attentive at first, but gradually began to be less available. "I couldn't blame them. I was bored and uncomfortable and miserable being with myself. It must have been even worse being in the room with me." She understood that they had their lives to live. "We were young, active, busy. But I expected my best friend to stick with me. That's what friends are about, isn't it? They're with you through thick and thin."

Yet this was not how it worked. Alysha's best friend, Sherry, virtually disappeared during Alysha's illness. "I had moved back in with my parents, since I could barely get myself to the bathroom and couldn't cook for myself. I was being taken care of physically, but I was really lonely. So I would call her, and we would chat for a little while. But even though she lived less than a mile away, she would never come over. I asked her if she was afraid of catching the illness, and she laughed like I was saying something stupid, but I knew some people were afraid that Lyme disease was contagious.

"What was amazing was that another friend totally stepped in for me," Alysha said. "Debra, the person who did show up, almost every day, was a true best friend. We hadn't been particularly close before that, but that didn't make any difference at all. Each time she came she brought me a magazine and a fruit smoothie and sat with me — usually just for a short time, maybe not even a half hour. I don't remember what we talked about — probably not anything of any importance. I was so tired, sometimes we wouldn't even talk, we would just watch something on TV, and then she would leave.

"She was there for me during those awful days. That's a good friend. Not just someone who is there when you need her, but someone who can figure out when to talk and when to just sit with you in silence. Sometimes it was just the idea that she was keeping me company. I will always be grateful. And if she ever needs anything from me, I'm there for her. I just hope that I'll be as good at it as she was."

A Friend Is Trustworthy, Honest, and Nonjudgmental

Knowing that a friend has your back in times of trouble means that you can trust her. But trust takes a number of different forms. One of those forms is mutual honesty, a sense that a friend will tell you the truth and that you can do the same for her. Honesty does not necessarily mean blurting out all of your unfiltered thoughts, but it does mean sometimes being willing to say things that your friend might not want to hear. And it means listening when a friend tells you something you don't like.

A fifty-seven-year-old artist captured this aspect of friendship beautifully. She said, "When my best friend told me that she thought I should get a hearing aid, I was really upset. I felt like she was saying that I was old, or that there was something wrong with me, and it really hurt my feelings. But because I trusted that her intentions were good, I asked a couple of other people. It turned out they were aware that I had been having troubles hearing, but hadn't wanted to distress me, so they didn't say anything. Now I have a really good hearing aid, and I'm grateful to my best friend for having the courage to tell me that I needed it."

Another woman said, "I have a friend who's my go-to person when I'm buying an outfit for an important event. She won't flatter me into buying something I don't look good in. She tells me the truth, even when I might not be completely comfortable with it. It's true about everything in our friendship. I don't always like what she says, but I always trust her to tell me the truth."

Mutual trust also means believing that your friend will not judge you for your failings and will not hurt you intentionally — and it means working hard to do the same for her.

A working mother in her mid-thirties, part of a group of friends who first met in elementary school, said, "I'm so lucky to have them. They've saved my marriage more than a few times, and I know I've done the same for them. We can talk about anything, and the best news is that we won't criticize each other for what we're feeling. That doesn't mean we don't criticize each other's behaviors sometimes, but we always know that it's with love. So when I'm really pissed off at my husband about something that he just doesn't understand, I can talk to my friends about it. I get whatever it is off my chest, and sometimes I get good advice. But I always get understanding. They always make me laugh about something — a lot of times at myself. But it's always with love, so I feel better, and that frees me to have a better relationship — as myself — with him."

She added, "It's really important that we trust each other to keep what we say inside the group. We don't gossip. If that trust wasn't there, none of the rest of it would work."

Room for Bad Feelings

Stephen Mitchell, the American psychologist and founder of the relational school of psychoanalysis, writes that we need different people to affirm different aspects of ourselves.[17] For Adeli and Richelle, some dissimilarities in their experiences made it easier for them to communicate their understanding of each other. Richelle could talk to Adeli about things she could not tell her sisters, who were basking in the glow of their own new families. But in part because Richelle did not have a baby, Adeli was comfortable sharing some of the difficulties she faced as a new mother with Richelle, more so than with her friends who seemed so happy and competent. "I can't believe how hard it is," she said. "It always looked so peaceful and lovely when I saw women with their babies in snugglies. That was what I was looking for. I feel like there's something wrong with me for complaining. I must be a terrible mother."

Despite her own aching desire for exactly that idyllic image, Richelle, who had supported her sisters through the early difficulties of parenthood, was sympathetic. "I told her that I had seen how hard it was, but that it looked to me like it gradually got easier." But what was also important for Richelle was what Adeli said when she revealed her inability to get pregnant. It turned out that Adeli had also had troubles getting pregnant. "Oh, it must be so hard for you to be around your sisters and their babies — and to be with me, here!" she said with compassion. "You must be so angry!" Richelle felt her pain reflected back to her in a way that actually helped. She could not explain it, she said, but there was something about her new friend's recognition and understanding that eased the hurt, just a little. She felt understood "from the inside," she said. In psychological language, she felt mirrored. Women are often good at being sympathetic and nurturing, but we do not always feel comfortable with our angry or negative feelings, and we therefore are not always comfortable reflecting those emotions back to other women. Adeli had given Richelle a gift by mirroring her anger with empathy and understanding, and without dismissing or sugarcoating it. Interestingly, Adeli also felt closer to Richelle as a result. Responding to a friend's need can make us feel more connected to them.

Different Friends for Different Needs

Many recent college grads spoke of the contrast between their friendships in college and those they were making as young working women. Those in their later twenties and early thirties seemed to have made a subtle shift toward less intense "best friendships."

"Really, now I just need to like a woman and feel as if we have some stuff in common to want to hang out with her," said one thirty-one-year-old. "I still have my old best friends from college. That'll never change. But I'm not looking for that kind of connection anymore. Actually, I wouldn't have time for it now anyway." Studies have found that this shift in what we need from our friends is a normal part of becoming adults. Women over thirty-five are less likely to see "understanding" as the central requirement of friendship.[18]

As we go through the different seasons of life, changing needs and expectations alter what we ask for from our friends. Many of the women I spoke with initially defined friendship with other women the way Kevin did — as a deep emotional connection. Yet when I asked if their ideas about friendship had changed over the years, even many of those who maintained close emotional ties with friends from college said that their ideas about what goes into friendship had shifted over time. In our twenties, we look for friends who will hang out with us, support us as we take the first steps toward adult life, and commiserate over relationship and work problems. As we move into our late twenties and thirties, many women settle into a career path, a more long-term relationship, and/or starting a family. Work friends are often different from friends with children, who are frequently not the same as friends we want to travel with, or those with whom we celebrate and mourn.

As we get older, our friendships often broaden and our expectations shift. We begin to include a wider range of women from different cultures and backgrounds. Age also becomes less significant. Many women spoke of the joy of mentoring younger women. Others told me of older women who had guided them through career choices and difficult periods in their lives.

Some long-term connections can survive life changes. One energetic fifty-four-year-old who had retired from her job as an office manager to babysit full-time for her three grandchildren said, "Most of my friends can't comprehend why I made the choice to take care of my son's children. Sometimes, even when I explain, they don't get it." She added, "I know I don't understand everything about them, either. But that doesn't stop us from being good friends."

Recognizing that no friend can meet all of your needs, nor can you meet all of hers, can help you negotiate the pain of disappointment when a friend is not there when you need her. Sometimes this means accepting that a friendship is over, as happened for Kelly, one of the "girls from Ames" whose forty-year friendship the author Jeffrey Zaslow describes in his book of the same name.[19] Zaslow writes, "The friendship ended over Kelly's disapproval of the woman's behavior and her inability to trust her." Accepting that this woman could not be the friend she wanted was both freeing and self-affirming.

But sometimes this moment of truth can deepen and enrich your friendship. Alysha, for example, found a different way of dealing with her own disappointment with her old friend Sherry. Months after recovering from her bout of Lyme disease, Alysha asked Sherry what had happened. "It turned out that she was afraid of my illness, not because she thought she might catch it, but because she was horrified by my helplessness. She told me that it was like I was someone else, and she didn't know what to say or how to be around me. She was deeply ashamed, but there wasn't anything she could have done about it.

"I learned something very important about friends," Alysha said. "No matter how much you love someone or how much they love you, they may not be able to be there for you when you need them. I realized that for me, part of being a good friend is to know what you can and can't expect from people, and not to expect more from someone than she can give you. I like to think I would have been there for Sherry, but the truth is, I'm not sure I could have, at least not the way Debra was for me."

Once she was healthy again, she and Debra grew apart. "She was a terrific caregiver. But I think she was more comfortable in that role than having me as a buddy to do things with. We went out a couple of times, but she couldn't stop trying to take care of me. When I asked her about it, she didn't seem to know what I was talking about.

"I care about her, and I'm grateful to her for what she did for me. But we are not as compatible as we were when I was sick and she was keeping me company. I think her strength is in taking care of people. It's what she likes best. And now that I'm healthy, I don't want to be taken care of. I want a more equal kind of connection. Maybe that's what made it hard for Sherry to be there for me when I was sick. She didn't like the inequality either. I guess one of the things about getting more mature is understanding that no one can be everything for you, and you can't be everything for someone else."

Are Social Media Friends
Real Friends?

And then there are the friends we make through social media.

Friendships in the cyberworld are defined in much the same way that friendships in the world of flesh and blood are. For instance, they often begin with shared interests and common experiences. A young professional woman who moved to a large metropolitan area for her first job after college said, "I had a lot of anxiety about finding new friends to replace my college friends. Starting out in a new city is really different from the mass desperation of freshman year, but it's kind of similar to the next few years of college. Everyone has settled into their friend groups, but you're still interested in branching out." She realized that she had made new friends in college by joining clubs, societies, and activities. It was harder to find an equivalent in the post-university world, but online she discovered that she could meet like-minded people in her city. "People will sometimes post about an activity that they want to do," she told me. "There were open invites for a variety of different things — like playing board games at a café, barhopping, or going for a hike with a new puppy." Numerous women find female partners online for a variety of activities, from jogging or tennis to writing and wine tasting. "I'm not 'best friends' with any of them, but some of them have definitely become friends," said one twenty-seven-year-old who got involved in a parks cleanup project through an online site that promotes volunteer activities in her city. "Sometimes we go out for coffee or dinner, or even to the movies or a concert. And some of them I just see when we're working at the park."

Culture and lifestyle differences have an impact on how we think and feel about social media and Internet friendships. Younger generations have grown up with these relationships and often take them for granted. Some older women find online connections a little unsettling, but many take advantage of technology to stay in touch.

Many women in their fifties and sixties told me of using social media to keep up with friends all over the world. Magdalena, a vibrant grandmother in her late fifties, talked about her best friend in elementary school. Living in a war-torn country in the Middle East as children, they had each moved away with their families when they were eleven. Yet somehow they managed to get occasional letters to each other. When they were in their late teens and again in their early twenties, Magdalena's friend had come for a long visit. Then marriage and growing families once again made it impossible for the two women to meet in person. For them, electronic media "is the best thing ever!" Now friends on Facebook, WhatsApp, and Instagram, they feel as though they are part of each other's lives. They share everything from photos of their homes, children, and grandchildren to family activities and "random thoughts." Private messaging and occasional phone calls allow them to discuss more personal topics. "The only thing that would be better would be if we lived close enough to visit regularly," Magdalena said.

There are, of course, potential dangers to cyber friendships. As one young woman put it, "You don't know who these people are. What if they turn out to be stalkers?"

A tired-looking woman in her fifties said, "I thought I had found my soulmate, but I just had my soul stolen." She had experienced "catfishing," a scam in which fake online friends tell touching but untrue stories of sick children, drug and alcohol problems, and financial difficulties in order to siphon money from unsuspecting online buddies. Such stories are not uncommon, according to recent reports, so it is important to be alert to these possibilities when making friends online.[20]

But social media can create rewarding and meaningful connections as well. A recent program on National Public Radio reported a group of teenage girls who developed a platform to use social media and online friends to build self-esteem and counteract online bullying of other girls.[21] They are clearly onto something important. Researchers have found that positive online experiences like the ones reported to me by so many women are a large part of today's world of friendship. Programs like Snapchat, Instagram, Twitter, Tumblr, Reddit, Pinterest, Vine, Kik, Pheed, Wanelo, 4chan, ASKfm, WhatsApp, GroupMe, iMessage, Periscope, Tinder, and Yik Yak (to name just a few) have been found to promote traditional kinds of friendships among women of all ages — despite the anxiety that even mentioning "social media" can cause some of us.[22]

Social media is also useful for reconnecting with old friends. Simply discovering someone we used to know is often as far as it goes. As the blogger Sara Coughlin writes, "Maybe some of us just like to keep up with that girl from high school who became a Fitspiration Instagram star, okay?"[23] But numerous women share stories of reconnecting with old classmates who go on to become new friends. As a forty-something named Drayaa said, "I went to my high school reunion with trepidation. I was afraid of people's judgment. And I came away with a new friend. A woman I had barely known in high school turns out to be one of the most interesting people I've met in a long, long time." Their history and knowledge of each other provided a base for the new link between them, but their adult friendship was based on who they were in their forties, not who they had been at sixteen. Living in different cities, they developed this new connection with the help of electronic communication. "It could never have happened without Facebook, FaceTime, and Instagram," Drayaa told me. "We get to see each other, even when we can't be in the same place. That's different from just talking on the phone, which we also do."

One of the things about social media friends is that they provide both companionship and boundaries. You don't have to stay on the phone or at the party when you're checking or chatting with a friend on Facebook or Instagram, or when you're texting or messaging. The boundaries are, to some extent, simply built in.

Companionship and Boundaries

Some women told me that they had no interest in the kind of close, intimate friendships that my friend Kevin envied. "I need my space," said one woman in her forties. "I like my independence," said another. And another told me she disliked the idea that someone might even think that they knew what she felt. "It seems too intrusive," she said, and added, "I'm a loner. I don't like groups, and I don't like opening myself up. And besides, how can anyone know what someone else feels?"

Yet many of these same women had friends they saw occasionally, women who were their "movie friends," for example. "We go to the movies once or twice a month," the woman who called herself a loner told me. "We actually don't like the same kinds of films, so we expand each other's horizons. One time we'll go to something I like, and the next we'll go to something she wants to see. But do you call that being friends?"

A professional woman in her sixties echoed the words of many others when she spoke of her expectations for herself as a friend. "For many years I believed I needed to be available anytime a friend needed something from me, whether it was to talk about her problems, share good news, or go for a walk or to a movie. I felt bad because I've never been that kind of woman. My husband was my best friend, and my kids and my work took most of my attention."

"But now that I'm retired and my children are gone, I have more time. I like the women I know, and I've started seeing more of them." She added, "I'll never be someone who goes away for a 'girls' weekend.' That's not me. But where I used to think I had to ignore my own needs in order to be a friend, now I see friendship differently. I can be a good friend without giving up all of my autonomy. I just have to be myself."

Lily, a lively eighty-seven-year-old who lives in a residential community, told me that her need for and definition of friendship had shifted. "Someone who can tell me an interesting story at lunch, or who will call and talk on the phone for a while is a friend," she said. "Most of us are in some kind of assisted living. I have old friends who still remember my parents or my husband. Sometimes talking to them is like looking through old photograph albums. But I also have a group of lunch friends, women I see most days in the dining room at our residence. We're a very mixed group. Our ages go from seventy-six to a hundred, and our backgrounds are all over the place. Some of us were married and some not, some have children and some don't, some of us worked and some of us were homemakers. We probably would never have been friends when we were younger. But we're fond of each other and we worry about each other. We save each other seats at our table. Other people want to join us, but we don't want them. I guess you could say we're the 'in group.' But we don't see one another except at lunch time." She smiled. "It's a perfect friendship. Not too intrusive, but connected just enough to make us feel both alive and not alone."

We all know that to have a friend, we need to be a friend. At that dinner when Kevin talked about wishing he could have friends like women do, he said, "My wife has those kinds of friendships," which prompted me to ask her if she could say what made her a good friend. She replied, "I think about my friends and want to know what's happening in their lives when I'm not with them."[24]

I have asked this question of many women. The answers range from "I listen to what my friends tell me and I remember the important things," to "I try to do little things for them, like remembering their birthdays," to "I don't know. I just like people, and they become my friends."

A twenty-nine-year-old banker said, "I try to stay in touch with my friends, even when I'm super-busy. It only takes a second to text someone to let them know you're thinking about them." A thirty-five-year-old working mother said, "My friends know that I'm thinking about them even when I don't have time to text them. We've been part of each other's lives for such a long time, we know the love is there even when we can't connect." And a thirty-eight-year-old waitress said, "I don't have time in my life for lots of drama. I cut my friends plenty of slack. When somebody does something I don't like, I tell her, but I know that in most cases she isn't doing it to hurt me. Nobody's perfect. To me, being a friend is accepting those imperfections."

A forty-two-year-old computer programmer told me, "When I get together with one friend, we talk about our feelings, and about things that have to do with our families — our kids, our husbands, our parents. But another friend and I never discuss anything personal. Our main connection is that we like to go to lectures at our local community center together. Being friends with her means sometimes going to a presentation I might not really care about and knowing that she'll do the same for me another time. It's kind of a give and take, although we don't keep score or anything like that. But we help each other to step outside our comfort zones from time to time. I enjoy learning new things with her, but I like that I'm being a good friend by helping her grow too."

A fifty-five-year-old lab technician said, "I've been thinking about this question a lot recently. For the last few years, while my marriage was falling apart, I stopped being a good friend. I was so focused on my own pain that I couldn't pay attention to anybody else's needs. Fortunately for me, the women I'm close to hung in there with me. Now that the divorce is over, and I'm feeling much better, I'm able to pay attention to what's going on in their lives. I'm sort of quietly trying to make up for my past self-involvement.

"But when I told my closest girlfriend that I was feeling guilty about having been so self-centered for the past few years, she said I was being crazy. She said I had been there when she needed me in the past, and I would again in the future. I guess that's what really defines being a friend for me. Being there for your friends when they need you, and letting them be there for you when you need them."

And a sixty-two-year-old told me, "I don't have a lot of friends. But I think one of the most important ways I'm a friend is to not be judgmental. My closest friend is obsessed with her own dress for her daughter's wedding, which she worries means she's being selfish. She says it's supposed to be all about her daughter, not her. I reminded her that wanting to look good at her daughter's wedding does not make her a terrible mother. I said it would be worse if she didn't care how she looked, or if she showed up in something that embarrassed her daughter. She just texted to thank me for all my support, but I think I should thank her instead. Being able to give her the backup she needs — well, that makes me feel good."

Connecting, in whatever way works for you, appears to be one of the keys to women's friendships. Going to the movies, taking a walk, pitching in when a friend is sick or in need, shopping for a special occasion, sending an occasional text, or just chatting about small, unimportant things are all ways that women connect with one another. These important relationships are not always simple, however. They can be troubling as well as rewarding. We will explore ways that you can be a better friend, sometimes by managing the difficulties differently or more effectively. Because *having* friends feels good, but *being* a friend can feel even nicer.

3

Friends and Family:
One We Choose, One We Don't

THERE IS A POPULAR SAYING THAT WE CHOOSE OUR friends, but not our family. This was certainly true for Janie, an actor with hair and makeup reminiscent of a young Liza Minnelli, who told me that her mother never had a nice word to say about anyone. "She didn't like her own friends, so how could she possibly like mine?" Janie said. "But still, she talked with those women whom she didn't like every single day of her life. What's that about?"

As a child, Janie was embarrassed to bring friends home from school because she was afraid that her mother would say something mean to them. But to her surprise, her friends loved her mother.

"They thought she was funny and smart. And they didn't mind it when she criticized them. It just didn't feel hurtful to them the way it did to me." Janie kept her friends away from her mother anyway. "I didn't want her telling me all the negative things she thought about them. I wasn't afraid that she would change how I felt about my friends. I just didn't want her near them."

As she got older, Janie had less and less contact with her mother. "She made my life miserable in many ways. I realized that my friends were much more supportive and loving than she was. My friends have become my family."

Like Janie, a number of the women who spoke with me said that they got most of the support, mirroring, and understanding they craved from friends, not family. Even women who were close to their families said that friends met many of their needs. A young college soccer player captured this split when she said, "I love my family, but I can't talk with them about anything meaningful. I have my friends for that."

Many women told me that their friends made life bearable at a time when their families were falling apart. The novelist Jay McInerney puts it this way: "The capacity for friendship is God's way of apologizing for our families."[1] "Holiday gatherings were so painful in my house," said an adult daughter of long-divorced parents, "that my siblings and I stopped going back years ago. I have a huge Thanksgiving dinner with friends every year — and the first thing I do when I wake up on Thanksgiving Day is to give thanks that those wonderful people are part of my life!"

Janie told me, "My best friend throughout my childhood lived a few houses down from us. I would go there almost every day after school, and I stayed for dinner more often than not. I learned about caring and connecting from that friend and her mom, from watching them interact with each other in ways that were so different from my mom's and mine. I absorbed this by osmosis, I think." Although Janie and her childhood friend grew apart, she said, "She will always have a special place in my heart. I don't think I would have become the person I am today if she had not been there when I was a child."

We learn first from family and later from friends how and when it is acceptable to express or even allow ourselves to have certain feelings. Friends teach us to manage feelings that our families are not particularly comfortable with. For instance, Juliana, a Vietnamese-born woman who was sent to boarding school in London as a young child, told me that she had never allowed herself to feel a wide range of emotions before she became close to her circle of adult women friends. "They opened up a world of feelings for me. And not just loving and caring ones, although those are so important! They have also taught me to be angry and selfish, and to feel loneliness and hurt. None of those feelings were okay in my family. And they certainly weren't okay in school. I grew up closing off all of my emotions. That was how I survived, you know?" She smiled with delight and added, "You still wouldn't call me someone who goes around with my feelings on my sleeve, but I feel like I used to live in the shadows, and now I live in a rich and colorful world of friendship!"

Many of the women I spoke with said something very different: family members were their best friends. Others told me that friends and family were equally important parts of their lives. In each of these instances, these women made it clear that connections in various forms are crucial to their happiness. This idea is a basic tenet of attachment and relational theories: we humans are biologically "programmed" to connect. The psychologist and neuroscientist Matthew Lieberman goes so far as to suggest that our need to be socially connected "is an evolutionary advantage that has been baked into our operating systems over millions of years."[2] It is, he tells us, what keeps us alive and makes life meaningful. So it would make sense that we would stay connected to our families when possible, even though we also develop friendships outside of the family circle.

Learning to Connect

Usually, our first significant relationships are with our parents, who provide our earliest models for connecting with others. Children learn as they simultaneously participate in and observe their family's particular styles of attachment. How our parents relate to us, of course, colors much of how we relate to others. But watching our parents interact with their own friends also has an impact. Many women told me that they had grown up admiring their mothers' friendships with other women and had tried to emulate them. "My mom and her girlfriends used to visit with each other a lot. They'd bring all the kids together and have morning coffee before they headed back to their own homes to do their housework or other tasks of the day," one woman in her sixties told me. "A lot of the kids would go off and play, but I loved sitting in the room with the women, listening to them tell stories and laugh. I got such a sense of peace when they were laughing, even though I usually didn't understand what they were talking about.

"Sometimes they cried too, and a lot of times they would pat each other on the hand," she said. "There was such a sense of solidarity between them. I told myself that when I grew up I would have friends like that. And I do. I have a wonderful, loving group of friends who've been part of my life since I was quite young. They are my support, my joy, and my solace."

By contrast, many women told me that their mothers were role models for how *not* to have friends. Preethi, a thirty-six-year-old radiologist, said, "Mother has a best friend she talks to every day. And every day she gets off the phone and lists all the things she doesn't like about this woman, who she calls her dearest friend." Preethi had therefore purposely developed a very different way of dealing with her friends. "I have lots of friends. It's not like I go looking for them, but they seem to find me. And when they do, I look for the good things about them. Nobody's perfect, but I focus on the positive, not on the negative."

Siblings are also important role models. How older brothers and sisters respond to us and our friends can influence our own feelings about our connections outside the family circle. "My big brother treated all of my girlfriends like just more little sisters," said one energetic personal trainer. "He was incredibly caring and gentle with all of us. I think that's probably a big reason why I'm so outgoing now."

Siblings often teach us about connecting to peers in ways that parents cannot. Richelle, who comes from a large family, said, "My brother has always been my idol. He's eighteen months older than me, and we were always together. I think I learned everything I know about being connected from him. I want to have a group of friends like he has. They've been together since high school. They're in their thirties now, and several of them are married and have kids. And still, they get together."

Younger siblings as well as older ones can teach us skills that will play a role in our friendships. Many women shared stories about rivalry with a younger brother or sister. They were often surprised when I asked if any of these issues had emerged in their friendships, and some could see no connections at all. But some women described links between their early sibling relationships and their adult friendships. For example, one engaging mother of five laughingly said, "When we were young my little sister and I would fight like wildcats. We would pull each other's hair and scratch each other till someone separated us. But we were also best friends. We loved each other desperately and were miserable when we were separated. I think she's the reason I have always been able to tell friends when they were doing something that upset me. I don't keep these things to myself, like some women I know do. I don't get into physical fights anymore, of course, but I'm not afraid of conflict. I know that I can be furious with someone I love. The bad feelings come and go, but the love is always there."

Friendfluence

Friends can also influence how we feel about our families. In Jeffrey Zaslow's book *The Girls from Ames,* ten women whose forty-year friendship began in grade school tell us that they shared relationships not only with one another, but also with one another's families.[3] The girls' families influenced their friendships, but their home life was also influenced by their friendships. While many psychologists today focus on the importance of family, and especially parents, in developing children's personalities, Erik Erikson, the psychologist who introduced the idea that psychosocial development goes on throughout the life cycle, would have applauded this insight. He believed that friends help children learn how to live in the world outside their family.[4]

Friendship experiences sometimes break old patterns of interacting that we have learned within our family, patterns that may have been handed down from our parents' parents to them and then to us. From very early in our emotional, psychological, and social development, friends introduce us to new ways of experiencing other people.

A friend's personality and style of interacting can activate aspects of our personality that may not be expressed at home. Juana is an example. An outgoing lab technician now in her early thirties, she told me that her mother had always been anxious and hovering. "She was afraid to let me climb on the jungle gym in the park when I was little, and she did not want me to walk to school with my friends as I got older. She was always worried that something bad would happen to me." Her dark eyes were serious when she said, "But my very best friend, Elyssa, came from a different kind of family. Her mom encouraged us to be adventurous. She told us that a scraped knee was nothing to worry about — that it would just make us strong! Elyssa was an adventurer, and I followed her lead. And, fortunately for me, her mother helped calm mine down. I would never have been allowed to go out of state to get my technical training without her support."

Research has shown that our brains react in distinctly different ways to different people.[5] This is one of the reasons that you can sometimes feel like you are not yourself, or at least not the self you are most comfortable with, when you are with certain people. For many women, as was true for Juana, the presence of a friend and that friend's family can encourage the development of sides of ourselves that our own family either cannot see or cannot support.

Friends also teach us about what have been called the "unwritten rules" of friendship,[6] which can be very different from the rules of relating we learn in our families. One mother of a toddler told me, "My daughter was biting other kids, and I couldn't figure out how to stop her. Nothing I did made a difference. And then one day one of the other kids bit her back, and that was the end of that!" Another mother of an eight-year-old said that her daughter had been showing off how well she could read, and one of her best friends said, "You hurt my feelings when you do that." This mother said, "My daughter was horrified. She hadn't realized that her behavior could have that kind of impact on her friend. I had mixed feelings about it. I want her to feel comfortable with being proud of herself, but I also want her to respect other people's feelings. It was a difficult lesson, but one that she will have to figure out over and over again."

Painful experiences can help us learn to interact in the world of relationships. At the best of times, families help us negotiate bumps in the path of friendship in a way that advances our ongoing psychological growth, and friends help us grow emotionally as they support us through family difficulties. But sometimes neither friends nor family smooth the way, and it can take time to overcome the pain and develop trust in others. Juliana did not blame her parents for sending her from her native Vietnam to boarding school in England. "They were trying to make sure I got the education and experience that they believed would make my life easier than theirs. It just wasn't in their knowledge base to think that separation from them at such a young age could have an emotional impact that was far more damaging to me than a lack of education would have been."

Then, when her best friend at school rejected her, Juliana withdrew into herself. It was not until the birth of her children, when she began to meet other mothers, that she suddenly realized that something crucial had been missing from her life. "The group of women I met after my children were born changed my life. They are my family, my support, my base. I am so grateful to have them around me."

My Mother (Partner, Child, Sister, Brother) Is My Best Friend

Different cultures have different views about separating from family. In some parts of the world, adult children are expected to remain closely involved with their biological family, while in other places it is common for a married couple to engage with one spouse's family while separating completely from the other's. In other parts of the world, however, separation from parents is seen as part of the process of growing up. Research has found that both age and cultural differences[7] influence our attitudes toward these connections. But among many of the women I spoke to, whatever the cultural expectations, there was frequently some confusion about boundaries, separateness, and intimacy.

For instance, a doctoral candidate in her late twenties said, "My mother is my best friend. My peers act like there's something wrong with that. I don't know. The thing is, I can talk about anything with her, even stuff I can't share with other women my age. Maybe there's something wrong with me for feeling that way. I don't feel like it's a problem. I have a boyfriend, a profession, and other friends. But I don't know. Maybe they're right. Maybe I'm stunted or something." The ever-popular television series *Gilmore Girls* explores some of the problems that confront a mother-daughter duo who are also best friends. Despite wishing they could be as close and open with their own mothers, daughters, and friends as Lorelai and Rory are with each other, many women are also distressed by the lack of boundaries between the two women. "It's almost like they don't know how to be separate," said one woman. And another said, "They're both narcissists who can only really love each other as much as themselves, since they're basically the same person."

Aurora, a fifty-three-year-old middle school teacher and practicing Muslim with two teens, was suffering from her mother's recent death. She was not conflicted about the close relationship she'd had with her mother. She said, "I have some very good friends at work and in my community. But my mother was the person who really *knew* me. She became ill a couple of years ago, and passed away last year. It has been a terrible time for me. We lived a couple of miles from each other, and although we each had our own busy life, I talked to her every day. She was close to my kids and my husband too. I still miss her. She left a big hole in my life."

Similarly, a number of women described a close connection to their daughters, echoing one mother who said, "My daughter is my very best friend in the world. I love her more than anything. We are very close." Other women expressed criticism of such mother-daughter closeness, but research has shown that in some cases these attachments are an important part of normal, healthy adult life, second only to romantic relationships in fulfilling attachment needs.[8]

Friendships between siblings seem less susceptible to societal judgment. Many women told me that their siblings, brothers as well as sisters, were their best friends. For instance, Teresa, the second of four children, said, "We've gotten even closer since our parents passed away. Two of us live in the same town, but the third has moved to Latin America, where our parents are from, with her husband. But we're still incredibly close."

Others shared that although they were fond of or even close to siblings, they did not consider them friends. "No friend would come into my house and take one of my sweaters without asking," said one woman with two sisters. "But my sisters wouldn't hesitate to do that." And of course, plenty feel like the woman who said, "I love my siblings, but I don't like them. I would not be friends with them."

Teresa said that she and her siblings had other friends, outside of the family. But while her sisters shared friends and socialized with many of the same women, they did not always approve of some her friendships. "I kind of adopt a lot of needy people, and they aren't always crazy about my 'adoptees.' When my kids grew up and left home, I needed somebody to take care of, and these friends are people who need me. They're grateful to me, so it makes me feel good, like I'm needed. So even though my siblings don't approve, I have these other connections. But I'm closest of all to my family."

Richelle, the young woman who idolized her older brother, struggled with infertility while her siblings were busy starting their families. She told me something that many other women shared. She said, "I love my brothers and sisters, but my family doesn't talk about hard stuff. Our parents didn't even live together, as a matter of fact, but we never ever spoke about it. I go to my friends to talk about feelings." When she was trying unsuccessfully to get pregnant, it was not her sisters who helped her with the pain. "They were all having babies, and I didn't want to rain on their parade. I was so sad and hurt and angry and envious — all rolled up into one ball of misery — and none of them seemed to have the slightest idea. My friend Adeli is the one who got it. She's the one who got me through those terrible years. Even my husband wasn't as much support. He was going through the same pain as me, but we couldn't always talk about it. Adeli was *always* sympathetic, and always ready to talk. She was also okay with not talking about it. She was happy to distract me, or to even pretend it wasn't an issue sometimes. She took her cues from me. That was different from my sisters, because I knew that even when Adeli and I weren't talking about it, she understood that the pain was always there for me. I didn't get that feeling from anyone in my family."

However, Richelle's close friendships wouldn't have been possible without some early lessons from her siblings. Like many women, Richelle told me that even though her siblings never spoke about the fact that their parents did not live together, they were always there for her when her father forgot a birthday or did not show up for an important school event. "I think I carried that feeling of connectedness into my relationships with friends," she said. "I just expected they'd be there. I think that's what I saw in my brother's friendships too. Just the feeling that they would always be there for each other."

Unfortunately, some of what we learn from siblings about connecting is painful. Women who had been hurt by siblings in childhood told me that they often found themselves expecting friends to hurt them as well. "It's just what people do," said one woman whose older sister had been particularly cruel to her. If you grew up with a sibling who was consistently hurtful, you might very well have come to expect that anyone who gets close to you will hurt you as well. Such an expectation can become what the psychologists Joseph Weiss and Harold Sampson call a "grim unconscious fantasy,"[9] that is, a belief about how others are going to behave, which you bring with you into any relationship. We do not question these beliefs. We simply accept them as reality.

Teresa, whose three siblings were her best friends, told me that she had learned how to be a friend from them. Yet another woman with three siblings said, "I assumed that everyone was always competing for attention, just like my siblings and I did. The loudest and most visible person was the one who got noticed in my family. So that's how I behaved with my peers. The person whose attention I wanted was always the adult — a teacher in school, a leader in some activity. Not a peer." In such cases, siblings set the stage for problematic friendships. But friends can also help undo these hurts and help us shift these patterns.

Daphne, for example, was almost forty and already had two children when she and her husband, Mike, adopted two siblings orphaned during a hurricane. "Life was a little crazy for a while," Daphne said. "But we were handling things."

Until she came home to find her best friend, Jennifer, in bed with Mike.

"It was awful," she said. "But I have to admit that I wasn't completely surprised. I grew up with siblings who often did mean things, completely out of the blue. I think that's why I became such a caretaker. I knew what it was like to be the one who got hurt. And I felt so sorry for that person." She thought that her children needed extra attention from her during the separation and divorce. Since she enjoyed spending time with them and loved hearing about their day, it never felt like a burden to her. Like working mothers everywhere, though, she had little time to spare for herself, and even less for her friends. "But my friends won't let me bury myself in my work or my kids. They arrange activities!" She stopped to laugh.

"It's really funny. They'll organize a movie day for all of the kids and the moms, and they'll insist I come. And then afterward, a couple of them will take the kids for pizza, and the others will take me back to someone's home for a glass of wine. They know I wouldn't come if they just asked me to, even though it's really exactly what I need. It's so hard to believe that I have friends like this!"

Numerous women told me that their spouse was their best friend, but that they sometimes worried that there was something wrong with this. One woman who worked as a paralegal and had teenage children said, "I think that I'm too tied to my husband. I mean, I'm a professional woman, and I could take care of myself and my children if something happened to him, but he's my best friend, the person I talk to about anything that's bothering me, and the person I want to do things with. So what would happen to me emotionally if he got sick or killed in a car accident? I don't like to think about it. Sometimes I make myself do things with other women even when I don't really care to, just to make sure that I have some connections — just in case, you know?"

Mara, who had recently married her longtime partner, Camila, said, "I could be happy if I never did anything with anyone else but her. She's my best friend, my partner, and my children's Mama. But Camila needs other friends. She's the most social person you ever met. We've found a pretty good balance, though. She gets me out of the house and out of myself in ways I would never do on my own; and I get her to stay home and nest sometimes, which she admits she loves, but wouldn't do without me."

In Sickness and in Health

Interestingly, there is evidence that some of the genes that play a role in our drive to make social connections are also connected to how our bodies manage illness and inflammation.[10] Apparently this is one of the ways that we are "programmed" to seek out connections. While we have seen that not all friends help in times of illness, in the best of situations, family and friends complement one another to help us cope when we are sick or injured — and their attention helps strengthen our immune system. A Duke University study found that among unmarried patients with coronary heart disease, 85 percent of those with close friends lived at least twice as long as those without these relationships.[11] And after reviewing the experiences of over nine thousand breast cancer patients, researchers at Kaiser Permanente in California found that ties to relatives and friends predicted a lower death rate among these patients as well.[12] Interestingly, researchers have found that stress and illness release "tend and befriend" chemicals in women, leading us to seek connection with others during these difficult times.[13] Not everyone wants company during times of stress, but if you do, it could be, at least in part, because of these messages that your body is sending to your mind.

The reasons for the higher survival rate are not completely clear, but connections to others have been shown to reduce both stress and depression, which can be factors in physical health. One cancer specialist suggests that these relationships offer some concrete benefits as well: "Having social ties may provide access to real assistance, like having someone to take you to the doctor or having someone to talk to about your concerns or to connect you with resources that can help you cope with the cancer."[14]

Aurora, the middle school teacher who was still mourning the loss of her mother, said that being connected to their religious community has played an important role in helping her get through this time of emotional and physical vulnerability. "I am tied to that community as well. The women who are my friends were also my mother's friends. They have helped me mourn and find ways to move on. I don't think I could have kept going without their support."

Suzanne was in her early thirties and working full time as an IT specialist when she got pregnant with her second child. "I was thrilled," she said. "My husband and I had been worried that we wouldn't be able to get pregnant right away, but it happened very quickly." But her life had changed, and so had her friendships. "A lot of my college friends were still single or had just gotten married. I was the first to get pregnant, and here I was, on my second child. And although I had friends at work, they weren't close." So when she miscarried in her third month, Suzanne felt that she had no one to turn to for support. "My mom was terrific. She told me about her own miscarriage, which I had never known about, and she said most of her friends had had one at some point as well." Suzanne's friends also stepped in to help. "I told one of my old college friends, and she called my mom to ask what she should do. And suddenly I had women I hadn't seen for a while coming over to take my toddler out to the park, or to get me out for a walk. It didn't take away the sadness, of course; but I felt so loved. It helped."

Lily, who lives in a residential community, also told me of family and friends working together. "I fell and broke my hip when I was in my early eighties. My children were great, but they don't live near me, so they couldn't get in to see me as often as they wanted. They called one of my friends and asked if she could organize some visitors for me while I was in rehab. Someone was there every day. They brought books and magazines, and food, which was a lifesaver, since who can get better by eating institutional food? And they would sit and chat for a little while, or just read while I rested or watched television. Nobody said anything about it, but I think they reported back to my children. When I was younger, I probably would have felt they were being controlling or invasive. But now, I like it that my family and my friends have this link. It makes me feel safe. As long as they don't start telling me what to do."

Adult Relationships with Friends and Family

As we go through life, we often have multiple opportunities for changing how we relate to brothers, sisters, and parents, but we may have difficulty taking advantage of these opportunities. Family members can often activate old and unpleasant feelings simply by walking into a room where we are standing. There is a neurological explanation for this phenomenon. Research tells us that our brains are triggered to return to old patterns when we experience familiar situations and faces,[15] so it makes sense that we feel our "old selves" emerge when we are in the presence of family. Friends can also activate these dormant aspects of our identity by behaving in ways that remind us of family members. Even in adulthood, friends can help us rework some of the automatic interactions that bring out parts of ourselves we would rather not see again.

For example, Eileen, who was now sister-in-law to her school friend Liz, said, "We don't spend all of our time with each other anymore. We have other friends, and of course I have my own family too. But we're all so connected that sometimes you can't tell who all the players are anymore, except by some of the physical differences. But I think we've all learned something from one another. Lizzie has a tendency to be bossy, like her mom," Eileen said, with a mischievous smile. "And I have a tendency to be kind of passive, more accepting. But being with her, watching her interact with her family, and learning from them how to stand up to Lizzie has helped me be more assertive with her and with my own brothers. And that's been great for our relationships — my brothers' and mine — and also for my relationship with Lizzie.

"I think some of that learning process has happened throughout the family. My husband, Lizzie's brother, likes to tease their parents that they are starting to look like my parents! That, of course, hasn't happened, but there's been a kind of intermingling, and some soft-ening on both sides. You can see it in some of the traditions too. My Russian-born Jewish grandma learned to make Southern fried chicken from a neighbor and taught it to my mom, who has now taught it to Lizzie's mother, who in turn showed Mom how to make Chinese wonton soup. I don't think Lizzie's mother has got-ten any less bossy, but my quiet, shy parents have become a little louder, a little more assertive, I think because of their friendship with Lizzie's parents.

"Our siblings are friends. And our children are not just cous-ins; they are very tight with one another. Friends from other parts of our lives get folded into the mix too. Colleagues from work, the children's school buddies, everybody comes together in some way or another eventually. For example, Lizzie's parents have a huge Chinese New Year celebration — it's a blast. They serve traditional Chinese foods, which they start preparing weeks in advance, press-ing all of the children, grandchildren, spouses, and anyone else who walks into the house into helping. But even though it's part of the tradition to complain, everybody loves it. I think most of our town is there for the actual meal."

What You Can Do

Most of us are not blessed with the easy interweaving of family and friends that Eileen described; but there are many possibilities for growth when you begin to think about some of the unsuspected connections between these two different groups of people in your life. Here's one important question to ask yourself: how do your family and friends activate and enhance your positive and negative feelings about yourself?

In an essay for *The New Yorker*, the author Rivka Galchen wrote that she and her mother "live two miles apart and can help or irritate one another at a moment's notice."[16] Daniel Goleman, author of the classic book *Emotional Intelligence,* tells us that one way to deactivate such automatic triggers is to physically move back from any situation that has stimulated old patterns that you don't want to engage in. For instance, you go home for a holiday celebration and immediately find that you are feeling put upon and neglected. Get out of the house, suggests Goleman.[17] Go for a walk. Or call a friend, whose voice and response to you will trigger other patterns in your brain. Wait until you have been able to find the self you want to bring into the interaction, and then you can try again.

Another solution is to bring a friend to family gatherings. Family therapists suggest that we all behave differently when there is an outsider present. Maybe that is the secret in Liz and Eileen's family!

When a *friend* starts to trigger old patterns of behavior that you thought you had abandoned, ask yourself if you have inadvertently found someone who arouses old feelings rooted in an earlier relationship. And then try to figure out how you might respond to this familiar pattern in a fresh new way. This is what happened for Janie, the Liza Minnelli look-alike whose mother was always criticizing her friends. "One day I heard myself saying something critical about my closest girlfriend. I realized I was sounding just like my mom. I don't want to be that kind of person, so I asked myself what was going on. Why was I suddenly being so picky?" It took a while, but Janie eventually realized that she was using criticism to protect herself from being hurt. "This friend had said something that hurt my feelings," Janie said. "I didn't realize it right away, but when I thought about it, I saw that I had been finding things wrong with her ever since then. My mother is very sensitive to even the slightest hint of criticism from someone else, and I started to see that nitpicking has been her way of protecting herself. She looks at the negative to sort of undo the hurt. But I don't think it works so well. You just keep getting hurt anyway."

Look for new ways to deal with negative stimuli. Often, this means not taking careless comments to heart, no matter how much they seem to be directed specifically at you. When Janie realized what had caused her negativity toward her friend, she did something that she said was "very different for me. I went to my friend and told her that she had hurt my feelings. I said, 'I don't think you meant to, and I don't think you even realized it, but this is what happened.' She was so amazing! She apologized immediately, and told me she could see why what she had said had hurt me. I don't know if it will work with my mom, but I'm going to try it on her. We'll see how that goes!"

Change often happens slowly, so don't give up when you do not get the positive results you are looking for right away. And keep in mind that both friends and family members can continue to teach you new patterns, just as you can teach new ones to them. Your job is to be open to these changes.

4

*Disillusionment, Betrayal,
and Rejection*

BEING DISILLUSIONED BY A FRIEND IS A NORMAL AND even expected part of growing up. Most of us had some experience of mean girls or fake friends, what the singer Tori Amos calls "cornflake girls," who sell out their best friends without a second thought. In fact, in one study 68 percent of the people interviewed had been betrayed by a friend at some point.[1]

The American Heritage Dictionary defines the word "betray" in several ways: "to be false or disloyal to"; "to divulge in a breach of confidence: betray a secret"; and "to lead astray; deceive."[2] Behavior based on self-interest, of course, is a normal part of life and can often be forgiven. But studies have found that a friend's betrayal is especially significant and almost always feels personal.³ Such betrayals frequently involve — or feel like they involve — some kind of rejection. Your friend has communicated that her own needs and interests come before yours; the message that hurts is that she does not care about you or value your relationship as much as you believed she did. This communication is what really destroys many relationships. It can also damage a person's self-esteem, self-confidence, and trust in others.

There are books galore about handling infidelity in a marriage. But what about when a friend is disloyal or unfaithful? Some of the women I spoke with told me that the loss of a friend was more painful than the loss of a lover. Julie Fitness, a psychologist who has studied and written about the impact of betrayal, puts it this way: "When those on whom we depend for love and support betray our trust, the feeling is like a stab at the heart that leaves us feeling unsafe, diminished, and alone."⁴ Just as friendships can promote physical and psychological health, even to the extent of strengthening the immune system, betrayal can cause more than emotional pain. In some cases it can bring on physical problems.⁵ The good news is that emotional pain, just like the headaches, back spasms, and even the cold or flu that you caught after you found out that a good friend had turned traitor, can eventually disappear. It will just take some work on your part.

When duplicity challenges friends in books and on screen, some kind of redemptive conversation often follows. In the popular show *Gilmore Girls,* a young mother and her daughter/best friend struggle repeatedly with feelings of disappointment, hurt, and disillusionment in their relationship, and their conciliatory talks are often both funny and honest. In a moving episode of *Orange Is the New Black,* two women in prison deepen their relationship and their mutual understanding after a series of painful betrayals.[6] But real life is often more like the dark struggles recounted in Elena Ferrante's fictional world. In the very beginning of *The Story of a New Name,* for instance, one of the main characters, also named Elena, betrays the confidence of her best friend, Lila, by reading a series of notebook diaries that her friend has left in her care. As often happens when a person reads someone else's private communications, Elena learns some things she would rather not have known, including what she felt was a lifelong betrayal by the other woman. "The more I read," Elena writes, "the more deceived I felt."[7]

These deceits happen more often than we might like, but to some extent they are simply part of the normal life process. For instance, many women in their twenties feel betrayed when a girlfriend gets caught up in a serious romantic relationship. As one recent college grad explained, "I'm truly happy that my best friend is going out with a terrific guy. But, and I know it's not rational, sometimes I do feel kind of abandoned by her. I mean, I've been there for her through all the dry times without a guy. It would be nice if she could still spend just a little bit of time with me now."

And there are those times when you are the one doing the betraying. You eagerly share a juicy piece of information with someone, only to realize, the minute it is out of your mouth, that you have just gossiped about one of your closest friends. Or you are the one who no longer has time for your college friends because you are totally caught up in your job, your love life, or your growing family. Have you turned into a mean girl?

Not necessarily. Whether you are the betrayer or the betrayed, the damage can sometimes be temporary, with the disruptions folded into the fabric of a relationship without too much destruction. Sometimes, however, the fallout can be permanent and life changing. In either case, how we interpret the rupture can add to or alleviate our pain.

When Betrayal Means Rejection

A betrayal can destroy a friendship when the combination of rejection and loss of trust are too great to overcome. Whether we find out that a friend has been talking about us behind our back or that she has divulged our personal or private information, hurt feelings can sometimes be healed, and sometimes not. A hospital nurse in her fifties told me, "I was in my late thirties when I found out that my best friend had been telling a third woman, someone we didn't know well, something I had shared in confidence. I survived the embarrassment of having my private information out in the world. But I couldn't be friends with her anymore. I knew I would never be able to trust her again."

Lies can also lead to loss of trust, although most of us can brush off a small white lie from a friend, especially when we understand that her motivation was to protect herself or someone else from discomfort or embarrassment. But when a lie hurts our feelings, it is harder to ignore. An executive assistant at a large insurance company told a story that captures how this can happen. "My best friend at work and I made a point of having dinner together every couple of weeks. It was a way to make sure we got a chance to connect away from the pressures of the job. One week Trina told me that she couldn't make our dinner because she had family in town. I totally got it.

"We weren't bound to any specific schedule, and her family, who she didn't see very often, definitely had priority over me. But when I got to work the day after our canceled dinner, one of our co-workers talked about what a nice dinner she had had at the restaurant where my friend and I were planning to meet. I don't know what made me suspicious — plenty of people go to that restaurant — but I asked what had made her choose that place. She sort of got evasive then, so I said, 'Oh, I bet you went with Trina. She loves that place!'

She turned bright red and mumbled something about having to get back to work."

Hurt, rejection, and anger are normal responses to this kind of deception. Similar feelings often emerge when you find out that a friend has been saying one thing to your face while doing or saying something completely different behind your back. Like Isabella in Jane Austen's *Northanger Abbey,* who blithely declares, "There is nothing I would not do for those who are really my friends"[8] to the best friend she is busy betraying, these so-called friends appear to lack any genuine care for your feelings.

This behavior hurts, but sometimes, what really stings is the sudden sense of being far less important to a particular friend than you thought you were. For Daphne, who discovered the affair between her husband, Mike, and her friend, Jennifer, one of the worst aspects of the experience was her loss of faith in her connection with two people who were very significant to her.

Daphne had always been a caretaker. Long before she had children of her own, she was the mom of her social group. "Some of my friends even used to send me Mother's Day cards," she said with a smile. Always what she called "a big kid," Daphne got used to the way adults and other children treated her as though she was older than her actual age. "I realized pretty young that I wasn't pretty or popular. But the pretty, popular girls came to me for soothing and support when their boyfriends dumped them or one of their group was mean to them or even when a teacher said something unkind."

She had, however, always been able to connect with one girl or woman who saw a more complete picture of who she was. Jennifer was one of those people. They met shortly after Daphne and Mike married and moved into the neighborhood where Jennifer lived with her second husband and their son. Daphne was used to being treated like "Dear Abby." "Many of my friends saw me as a shoulder to lean on. I was someone who could give advice and listen to problems, but did not have any needs of her own." But Jen was different.

"From the beginning," Daphne said, "she treated me like *I* was the younger sister. She offered advice, brought me chicken soup when I was sick, and helped me find childcare when my kids were little. I felt different about myself when I was with her. More like a whole person. It was like Jen saw all of the different parts of me. Or at least she acted as though she did, anyway."

The Rug from Under Your Feet

Like Daphne, many women spoke of feeling as though the rug had been pulled out from under their feet after a betrayal. They felt that they could no longer trust their friend, but that loss of faith spread beyond the betrayal: they also lost a sense of certainty about their own perceptions. "How could I not have known this was going on?" is a common question asked after a friend's deceptive behavior has been revealed. "How could I have trusted her?"

Jo, a successful professional in her late forties, told me that her world had been shaken when a good friend secretly went after a job Jo had been working toward for months. "It would have been hard enough if she had told me about it," Jo said. "I mean, she knew it was something I really, really wanted. But at least if she had been aboveboard, we could have talked and I could have dealt with it. Ours is a very competitive business, and I knew she was as eager to move up as I was. But she didn't tell me. She left me to find out from my boss. That really hurt."

A friend's betrayal can leave you wondering about everything she has done or said in the past: was it actually what it seemed? The duplicity can shift how you look not just at her, but at almost everyone you know. Robert Stolorow,[9] a psychoanalyst and philosopher, says this loss of trust is one of the worst things about any kind of trauma, and a betrayal can definitely be traumatic. You can, says Stolorow, end up feeling as if no one can understand what you are going through, that somehow you have moved outside the human experience.

The betrayal by the two people she trusted most in the world left Daphne feeling lost and alone. "I'm not sure I will ever trust anyone again," she said. The behavior melted the glue that held her life together. While she was trying to recover her own balance, she also wanted to make sure that her children did not suffer too much. "Their lives were changing completely," she said. Still, in some ways, that part was easy for her. "I'm a caretaker. That's what I do best. I figured it out so that the kids still got taken care of." Mike, who had moved out and was living with Jennifer, was still an integral part of the children's lives. "Even if he didn't love me, he loved them," she said. "So we worked it out so that he was there for them." But Jennifer had also been an important part of their lives, and they, like Daphne, now had to deal with the change in Jennifer's relationship with their mother. Now that Jennifer and Mike were together, the kids saw Jennifer when they spent time with their father, but they were well aware of her absence in Daphne's life.

"It was hard for them. We didn't want to tell them what had happened, but it was almost impossible to come up with a story they could believe. And I didn't want to lie to them. I'd had enough lies and deceit in my life!"

Someone to Blame

Daphne was tempted to blame Jennifer for the destruction of her marriage. In psychological terms, this singling out of one culpable person is called "splitting" — separating people and events into two categories, "all good" and "all bad." This psychological defense is one of the ways that we try to protect ourselves from intolerable or overwhelming feelings.

Research shows that despite changes in attitudes toward women in many cultures, many of us are still uncomfortable with feelings like anger and resentment.[10] Women also tend to avoid conflict, in part because we are afraid that revealing our difficult emotions will drive our friends and loved ones away. But when a friendship is disrupted by a friend's betrayal, we cannot avoid these painful feelings. We have to find a way to deal with emotions traditionally viewed as "unfeminine." For instance, you might feel bad about yourself for having them. Then, in order to protect your already damaged self-esteem, you try to keep anger and resentment out of your emotional bloodstream, inadvertently turning them into something else. Oddly enough, you could feel better experiencing yourself as a victim or a martyr rather than as an angry female; as the suffering friend who has been cruelly treated, you can at least feel womanly and expect that others might feel sympathy for you. You might then even be able to feel and express an allowable variant of a so-called negative emotion: self-righteous anger.

Thus, unwittingly, you have split the players in the situation into "all good" and "all bad."

Fragile psyches can experience almost any incident, even an apparently insignificant one, as potentially overwhelming. Some people, often those diagnosed with borderline personality disorder, tend to "split" like this frequently. But all of us do so at some point, especially when we are feeling injured or overwhelmed. In a marriage or a friendship, splitting can also allow you to jettison one person in order to maintain a connection to another. If Daphne had seen Jennifer as having seduced an innocent Mike, for instance, she might have been able to maintain and more easily repair her marriage and her self-esteem.

Although placing blame like this can be temporarily soothing, it has several negative consequences. For one thing, it leaves you with no explanation for your own mixed feelings. How could Daphne try to understand all the years of closeness to Jennifer if she turned her into a one-dimensional negative cutout, for instance? Also, splitting leaves you without a healthy way of processing the uncomfortable feelings that are part of any ongoing relationship.

It May Not Be Not What It Seems

One way to manage splitting is to recognize that sometimes a betrayal is not exactly what we perceive it to be, whether we are the offended or the offender. A clinical social worker in her late thirties told me that she had lost a close friend over a misunderstanding. "We had made plans to get together with our husbands. It was a complicated arrangement because everybody wanted to do something different. She and I finally came up with what we thought was a compromise, but when the time came to get together, my husband balked. He said I hadn't told him what we were doing and he didn't want to do it. We fought over it, but finally I caved and we canceled at the last minute.

"I was embarrassed and didn't handle it well at all. That was definitely my fault. But my friend got so upset. Her feelings were hurt; I understood that. But even after I took the blame and apologized, she couldn't let it go. After a while, I got mad, although I didn't say anything to her. I just pulled away. I decided that it wasn't worth the trouble to try to repair the friendship. I just couldn't keep being friends with someone who couldn't cut me any slack."

We know that friendships are often made around shared life events, but those events can also lead to hurt feelings. One successful, attractive single businesswoman said, "I've been to so many weddings and so many baby namings that I can't even count them. But none of these friends seems to think it might be nice to do something meaningful for me. Of course, they'll all happily show up at my wedding — if that ever happens. But I need a little loving attention now, not just sometime in the distant future. And that doesn't occur to them." Many other women echoed her words.

Not only changes in life situation, but also in personality, can threaten friendships, particularly as women get older. Problems occur when we take these changes personally, interpreting behaviors that are really not about us as though they are a betrayal. For example, Roberta was a spry octogenarian who had always been painfully shy. She told me that her outgoing best friend for most of her adolescence, Donna, paved the way for her in all social situations. "I went with her to church, to her family's club, and to Brownies and then Girl Scouts." But as they got older, Donna, always the life of the party, became a heavy drinker.

"At first it was just part of who she was, you know. 'Donna got drunk again last night, but wasn't she just wonderful dancing with every guy at the party?' But after a while, I didn't enjoy being around her. I knew that she would forget anything we talked about when she was drunk. She wasn't the same person anymore. I tried to get her to go for help, and she would say that she would. I even said I would go to Alcoholics Anonymous with her. She agreed to go with me, but anytime I brought it up, she said it wasn't a good time. I felt like she was just yessing me to death. She didn't care about me. All she could think about was what she wanted to do."

Donna had a problem, and like many people, she was unable or unwilling to do anything about it. Roberta's feelings of disappointment and frustration were understandable. But Roberta took the behavior personally. Donna's refusal to accept Roberta's offers of help felt like a rejection. And yet now, at the age of eighty-nine, Roberta understood what had happened in a different way. She said, "Donna had many problems in her life. She also came from a long line of alcoholics. I doubt there was anything more I could have done for her, but I wish I hadn't spent so much time thinking she was doing something to me. It wasn't about me at all."

Forgiveness and Vengeance

Many cultures consider forgiveness a highly moral and therefore valued act. The psychologist Harriet Lerner writes that a heartfelt apology can reaffirm a meaningful connection.[11] Yet mental health professionals often come across situations in which forgiving does not seem the healthiest way to deal with a betrayal.[12] Lerner and Jeanne Safer agree that while sometimes it is good to forgive and move on, sometimes it is better *not* to forgive, if doing so means ignoring or refusing to come to grips with the pain and hurt caused by the betrayal.[13]

The impulse to forgive is one way of trying to find closure. "Let it go," we tell ourselves. But when we try to do it before we are psychologically ready, it can feel false to us and to the person we are supposedly letting off the hook. And it does not lead to genuine closure.

This is what happened for Daphne. At first, trying to reconcile herself with both Mike and Jennifer, she told herself that she understood that what they'd done was an impulse of the moment, and that they were both terribly ashamed and sorry. She felt that she could be "bigger than all of that" and not hold on to her hurt and anger. But it was clear that this was not a momentary glitch. One day, after Mike had moved in with Jen, one of Daphne's children spilled milk on the kitchen floor. She lost her temper. "It wasn't like me," she said. "I don't usually get rattled by something like that, and I don't yell at my kids unless they've done something really, really bad." She realized that she was taking out her negative feelings on the wrong person. "I hadn't forgiven either Jen or Mike, and it was time to acknowledge it. But at least I was moving on from feeling hurt. Now I was just plain angry."

Anger is a normal and healthy stage in the work of letting go, but it too is not the end of the road. For many women, anger is harder to process than sorrow, and conflict is painful to acknowledge. It can help to know that owning these difficult emotions can allow you to move on from them.

Both hurt and anger can lead to a desire for revenge. Vengeance has, in some times and places, been viewed as an act of supreme loyalty; it has also been considered a sin. In an act of revenge, the betrayed becomes the betrayer. Revenge may feel good, but it seldom resolves the feelings caused by the original treachery.[14] Instead, retaliation can escalate all of the hurt, anger, and misunderstanding experienced on both sides, creating far more difficulty. Trying to understand the other person's suffering — how the whole situation appears according to that person's point of view — can sometimes help. Interestingly, studies have shown that the two parties involved in a betrayal measure the pain differently. The one who was injured, according to these studies, may experience the pain as significantly greater than the betrayer believes the betrayed one really felt. Turning away from revenge, as the Stanford psychologist Frederic Luskin reminds us, does not mean ignoring the pain, hurt, or anger caused by a betrayal. What it does, he says, is allow us to move on in a psychologically healthy manner.[15]

When Daphne finally came to grips with her pain and anger, she decided that she needed to break off contact with both Jen and Mike. "Maybe I'll really be able to forgive them someday. But for now, I need to own that I don't want to have anything to do with either of them." Of course, this separation from Jen and Mike was complicated by their involvement with the children. At first, Daphne had wanted to forbid Jennifer any contact with the kids, but later she realized that this wish was impractical and seemed vengeful. "It wasn't fair to the kids," she said. "It also made my life more complicated." She honored her own wishes and her children's by using email to make arrangements with Jen and Mike for activities and visits with the kids. "That way I also always had a record of what they promised and what time they said they would be there for the kids." Daphne explained to her children that "Daddy and Jen and I don't get along anymore, but they both still love you, and you still love them. So you'll keep doing things with them, just without me." Telling them more, she said, would have put them in a terrible position. "It might get me my revenge, but at what cost to them? I wasn't willing to do that to my children."

What You Can Do

Once you have faced the painful truth of a betrayal and your own feelings about it, you can start to process the emotions — the good, the bad, and the ugly. Sometimes the person who betrayed you is present to process those feelings with you. In that case, it can be healing to talk about what happened. But sometimes she cannot join you in that work, or you may not want to open yourself to the possibility of further injury, and that is okay too. The same is true when you have done the betraying. If your genuine apologies are not accepted, you may feel hurt and frustrated. In either case, you can still express your feelings, but maybe not to that particular friend. It is also perfectly okay if you want to act as if things are fine and you want your friend to do the same, although this solution works best when it works for both of you. Like Lillian on the show *Bridesmaids,* you might just want to say, "Why can't you be happy for me and then go home and talk about me behind my back like a normal person?"

In other words, there is no single right way to handle a betrayal, and it can be difficult to decide how you want to move forward. Whatever your situation, it is crucial to recognize and acknowledge, at least to yourself, what you are feeling. Putting the emotions into words can help you make a start in coping with the experience. Talking out what happened with the friend who is involved may be the optimal approach, though perhaps the most difficult. Such conversations, however, don't always make things better. Sometimes they aren't the best solution.

Although you may feel that you need to take immediate action, it is often smart to allow yourself a cooling-off period before choosing a plan. Sit with your feelings, and consider different options as they come to your mind. It's okay to daydream about revenge, but imagine other scenarios as well. Then think about what it would really be like to go forward with each possible response. Talking this out with someone you trust can help — though you may hesitate, wondering whether such a conversation might amount to gossiping or even taking revenge. Asking another person not to simply take your side, but to help you think about what might have motivated your friend and how to understand the broader picture, is not mean. And widening your perspective in this way often makes it easier to decide what you want to do — or not do — about the situation.

Of course, as discussed throughout this chapter, after a betrayal, you will very likely have to manage a number of emotions. Your feelings about what happened are not going to remain static. Hurt may turn into anger, or vice versa. And in some cases, anger may eventually morph into understanding and sometimes even relief. Each phase will require different emotional and maybe even physical responses on your part. The key is to stay as honest with yourself as you can — and, when possible, to explain your thinking to the people who are important to you. Sometimes, although not always, this will include the person who hurt you.

Remembering that betrayal may not be what it seems is another important tool. This can mean trying not to take the hurtful actions personally, even when it seems that you are the intended victim. As Roberta realized about Donna, the behavior may concern your friend's inner demons, not her feelings about you. It might seem that a friend intentionally hurt you when she was not thinking about you at all. Of course, her lack of consideration of your needs could be hurtful in and of itself, and you do have to deal with that.

Time also changes our sensitivity to a betrayal. Roberta, energetic and alert at the age of eighty-nine, told me that she still thinks about Donna. But she said, "I have different kinds of friends these days. Many of my oldest friends are in assisted living, or have died. The ones who are still living don't tend to get around, or don't remember anything, or don't have anything to talk about." She has become friendly with women younger than herself—women in their sixties, seventies, and early eighties. "They read and talk about interesting books, go to concerts and the theater, and are simply more involved in life," she continues. Some are the grown children of old friends, and others are friends of her own children. "When I was young, I never would have been friends with some of these women," she says. "Partly because I was too shy, and partly because I was too much of a snob. Donna, with all of her problems, was not only my entrée into social situations, but she was a mirror image of me in many ways. We came from the same background and went to the same church. These days some of my best friends are women with completely different backgrounds from me, completely different worlds even. But they are wonderful. And far from being shy, I'm sometimes the most talkative member of the group. It's a different me!" Roberta's enlarged world of friendships has made her less sensitive to the hurt caused by Donna.

Finally, there is one step that we all need to take in order to move on after a friend's betrayal. This one is often the hardest of all. After you have allowed yourself to feel and process your hurt, anger, and resentment, you will need to honestly evaluate your own role in the betrayal. *This does not mean that you are at fault.* But since a friend's betrayal happens in the context of a relationship, and since you were part of that relationship, it is likely that you were in some small way, perhaps a very subtle or extremely tangential way, also involved in what happened.

When Daphne finally did start to recognize the complex factors that had ended with Jennifer and Mike together in her bed, she said, "I didn't want to look at the painful truth of what had been happening in either relationship. Jen had been letting me know that she was miserable in her marriage and worried that her husband was having an affair. But I was totally caught up in my life with my new family. I told myself I didn't want to listen to something that would bring me down. But I was ignoring another fact, which was that Mike and I hadn't been happy for a while.

"I hadn't put it into words, but I was hoping that adopting the two children would bring us closer together. I didn't pay attention when he said he wasn't sure it was a good idea. He tried to remind me about some of the difficulties we'd had when our first two kids were little, but I didn't listen. I didn't want to hear."

It was not Daphne's fault that her best friend slept with her husband. But, she said, "Once I figured that part out, I could understand on some level why they did it in our bedroom. On some hidden level, probably without knowing it at all, I think they wanted me to see. It was an act of desperation *and* anger. They were both used to me being the nurturing one, and I was suddenly unavailable to either of them. So they made their needs known, loud and clear, in a way that I couldn't possibly miss."

Daphne's insight did not lead to a reconciliation with either Mike or Jennifer, since she felt that she could still not trust either of them to "use their words" instead of actions to let her know what was going on with them. But her insight did make it possible for her to move on. Several years later she was on speaking terms, albeit not particularly cordial ones, with both Jennifer and Mike. Daphne had remarried and had made new friends. "I know this is a little crazy," she said, "but I think they did me a favor. I decided it was time for me to stop seeing myself as only one thing. I am a nurturer, but I'm a lot of other things too. They made me look at who I really am and who I want to be, and that has made me so much happier to-day than I was then."

To reiterate, discerning the part you played, however minor, in this kind of rupture is not about blaming yourself — but it can have some important benefits. Understanding how you might have un-intentionally triggered some of the feelings that led to the behav-ior can actually eliminate some of the pain. And paradoxically, once you understand the multiple causes of the thoughtless or hurtful behavior, it may be easier to stop taking it personally.

You can let yourself off the hook. You might even be able to let your old friend off the hook. Or not. Either way, you will be ready to move on.

5

⌒

The Joy of Belonging,
the Pain of Exclusion:
Groups, Clubs, and Cliques

YNDI, A SCHOOLTEACHER IN HER FORTIES, WAS
one of many women who told me that she had never been
part of a group of women friends. "I've always looked at
those groups of women who have known each other since high
school or college, and who get together for a girls' weekend or night
out, and I've always kind of wished I could have been part of one of
those groups. But I'm just not that kind of person."

Her mother, however, was a different story. "Mom has always
had a group of women friends," Cyndi told me. "More than one
group, in fact. She has her Bible study group, her crafts group, and
her Christmas cookie exchange group. But there is also a group of

women she has known since she got married — she didn't go to college, so I guess in some ways this is her equivalent of those 'best friends since college' groups.

"She and my dad were close friends with all of these women and their husbands. My siblings and I grew up with their kids. We used to go away on vacations together, the whole big group of us. Most of us kids have grown apart, but the moms are still very close. They're in their seventies now, and they don't get together the way they used to. A couple of them are divorced and a couple are widows. Some have moved away, but they still can talk on the phone for hours, and once a year they try to get together for a weekend. I don't know how much longer they can do it, but it's kind of amazing. And wonderful. I think it must be just the best thing to have a group of friends like that."

What Makes a Group?

What makes some of us develop a lifelong group of friends and some of us not? To answer this question, we must first define "group." Technically, a group is "two or more individuals who are connected by and within social relationships."[1] Researchers who study group dynamics tell us that a meaningful group differs from one that comes together to take a test or hear a lecture or see a movie, in two important ways. First, a meaningful group has a mutuality in which each person influences and is influenced by the relational interactions within the group. And second, the group itself takes on a personality that is bigger than any of the individuals within it and can have an impact on each of the group members. Thus, we are often drawn to a group because of its personality or public persona. For instance, a group can give us status or make us feel good about ourselves — as in a sorority, or an organization that is providing a service to others. Alice, a seventy-year-old grandmother, connected with other grandmothers to read to children in an urban pre-kindergarten. She said, "I have made some wonderful friends from this group. At first we started getting together to choose books to read; and then we started meeting regularly to talk about other services we could provide. We've become very close. The women in the group are special, and I feel special being part of it."

But what makes some of us gravitate to a large group and some not?

Researchers have found that most of us are more comfortable with small groups than with large ones, which could explain why large groups often naturally break down into smaller clusters. Family experience can play a role, although the impact may be different in every case. For example, some women who grow up in families with large circles of friends are drawn to large groups themselves; but others, like Cyndi, prefer groups of two or three instead of the big gatherings with which she grew up.

Nila, an only child, told me that she had always had a large group of friends. "And now that I'm married, my husband and his friends have become part of that group. We are a mix of singles and couples, and now babies and children. We all go to one another's weddings and baby namings, of course, but we also vacation together — well, not all of us, but groups of us — and we get together to have dinner, go the park with the children, attend concerts, and anything else. For me, these are the brothers and sisters I didn't have growing up. I love this group!" Yet Tamar, also an only child, told me that she did not feel comfortable in large groups. "How can you have an intimate conversation with ten women? Or even five? I like being able to talk and listen and stay on topic, and you can't do that in a group."

Recent research[2] suggests that the way our brains are constructed plays an important role in these choices. Neurological imaging shows that some brains are more quickly activated by multiple social interactions, while others are more engaged by relating one on one or even by being nonsocial.

But even those women who are "wired" to enjoy groups are not always able to engage in a group situation without a little assistance. Sofia, a soft-spoken woman from South America, told me that she had always been a little shy. "But I had a friend, Valeria, who was outgoing and had a million friends. She brought me into her circle. And then I was friends with all of the other girls, and I was part of the group. Our friendship has lasted forever. We brought our boyfriends, and then our husbands and our children into the group. And our children are friends, not just with one another, but with all of the adults too."

Cyndi's mother, Mary, told me, "I don't think of myself as a 'group person.' It's just that I like people, and I like being *with* people. My friends and I have a good time together. We love to tell stories and we love to laugh. So when we get together, whether it's to do our handiwork or for our holiday cookie exchange, we do a lot of talking and a lot of laughing."

But, she adds, her groups have been a great source of support and solace as well. "When my husband died, there were all of my friends, from all of my groups, hugging me and praying for me. They brought food for my children and me to eat, took our dirty clothes home to wash, and took the children off for activities with their own families. I was in such a daze, I didn't even realize what they were doing; but looking back, I don't know how I would have gotten through that time without them."

Many of the women whose stories I collected believed, like my friend Kevin, that women have a capacity for a closer, more intimate bond than men do. A group of women is assumed to be mutually supportive, loving, caring, and nurturing. Some research suggests that in certain cultures that require women to live in closer contact, they learn to manage some of the more unpleasant aspects of relational life, such as anger, competition, envy, and jealousy. These women seem more comfortable with these dynamics than women in settings that encourage them to be more autonomous.[3]

Salma, a Muslim woman in her forties, told me, "I was very lucky to grow up in a world where women are often together. My women friends have always been my support. Of course, we do gossip, and we can say mean things and hurt one another's feelings. But when something is wrong, we know we can go to the women in our life for caring and healing." Salma said that she and her friends did not need a "girls' weekend" because they were together so often. "We have tea together a few times a week. We talk about our children, our husbands, our parents. A few years ago some of us decided that we wanted to stretch our brains a bit — we'd all gone to college, and some of us had jobs and professions, but we didn't have a lot of time to take classes or do anything intellectual. So we started reading. Our husbands were pretty supportive. Mine wanted to read some of the things we were reading, and he talked with some of his friends about starting their own reading group. It was pretty funny." She smiled. "We were reading biographies of famous women. And the men started reading books about the stock market. And then we got hold of one of their books, and we started learning about making investments. We were not major players, but we made a little money. And we had fun!"

Alexandra, who came to the United States from China, found some confusing paradoxes when comparing the relationships between women in the two cultures. In China, she said, "Women do not support one another so much. There's a lot of criticism and negativity. It seemed like Americans were so much quicker to make friends. They were so much more open. When I went back to China, it was like running into a brick wall. But I realized over time that you can eventually make close friends in China too. It just takes a bit longer. In the United States it goes so much faster, but sometimes it's not so deep. It's just a kind of friendly attitude, but not a deep connection."

Yet paradoxes exist even within cultures. Violet, a twenty-seven-year-old, almost lost a friend who turned into a "Bridezilla" during preparations for her wedding. Despite this near upset, Violet told me that her group of women friends was all-important. "We support each other on the big things and on the little unimportant ones too."

Why Cliques?

Groups are sometimes created for reasons that are not so positive and affirming, of course. Think about the beloved movie classics *Mean Girls* and *Clueless,* the pink girls in *Grease,* or almost any scene from *Heathers.* There is also the UK's *Tamara Drewe* and *Absolutely Fabulous,* Argentina's politically disturbing *Cautiva,* Spain's *Princesa,* and China's *A Simple Life* and *The Way We Are.* Although mean girls do not always grow up to be mean women, at times a group is used to protect and promote those inside it while rejecting the outsiders.

Many of the women with whom I spoke were left out of the "popular" group or some other clique when they were young. Some described the pain of being shoved out of a small clique that had once welcomed them. Others talked about how their skin color, family background, or religion made them a target of peers' hostility and abuse while growing up. Sometimes they were rejected for no clear reason at all.

Many women's groups have a hierarchy, often with one woman as the "head," or leader. Research shows that as long as the other women accept the hierarchy, although not always without complaint, the group can manage any difficulties.[4] But sometimes part of a group's identity is whom it excludes. Being rejected from such a group can have a lasting impact on how we feel about ourselves and how safe we feel with other women in any season of life.

For instance, Juliana, the dark-haired beauty in her fifties who had been sent from her home in Vietnam to boarding school in England, told me that her painful experience with girls in her boarding school was one of the reasons she kept a distance from other girls and women for so long. In her school, she said, there was a definite sense that light skin was better than dark, that round eyes were better than almond-shaped ones, and that unaccented English was the superior language. "I felt so left out and unwanted that I figured I was better off staying completely to myself." Numerous other women of a wide range of ethnic groups and physical characteristics talked about similar experiences. Dayana, who came from an island in the Caribbean, and Tawana, who was from an African country, were among many women who described being excluded from groups because their skin was too dark. "It wasn't just the white women who kept me out," Dayana said. "Black women too. You were acceptable only if you had light skin."

This feeling of being unwanted may explain the findings of several studies: members of minority groups tend to seek out friends among their own group. These friendships help foster a sense of identity and increase self-esteem.[5] Of course, when such close-knit groups reject other possible members, the cycle of insecurity and loneliness is reinforced.

"Mommy cliques," which many, many women told me about, are just one example of a throwback to childhood experiences with rejection and "mean girls." Nancy, a cheerful and outgoing young woman who generally has no difficulty making friends, told me of trying to join a group of mothers at her son's new school. "I don't know if I wasn't wearing the right clothes or if I had spinach on my teeth or my breath smelled bad," she said. "But they were not interested in being friends. They couldn't even make the effort to be friendly. And they clearly also wanted me to know that I was being left out. They kept making plans to get together with their kids without me, in front of me."

Kwame Alexander, an author of young adult books, says that the rage, hatred, and murder we are struggling with in our world today "is not new. I would like to believe that the children are going to be able to have a better world."[6] But, he continues, if we adults don't give them the tools, they will not connect with people who don't look like them, don't sound like them, and don't think like them.

Fairy tales and science fiction often explore failures to connect with those who seem "other." In these stories, the outcomes can be cruel and the lessons learned painful. In her book *Uprooted,* Naomi Novik,[7] author of the critically acclaimed Temeraire novels, explores the question of why we hate others for being different. She suggests that good people lose sight of their own values or the truth of others' humanity because of the need to blame someone for bad things that have happened.

The psychologist Melanie Suchet writes that the desire to hurt someone else often comes from a feeling of having been injured oneself.[8] And one of my favorite psychoanalytic writers, Heinz Kohut,[9] says much the same thing. Cruelty, he tells us, is often a reaction to feeling injured, either physically or emotionally. It is a way of repairing damaged self-esteem that has made us feel weak and vulnerable.

The psychologist Erik Erikson explains that sometimes such prejudice is the result of incomplete identity development.[10] Identifying with an "in-group," or a group that shares your interests and excludes others, is a psychological defense against feeling confused about your own identity. Being part of the in-group can help build a sense of self. As the *Psychology Today* columnist Carlin Flora writes, "The right group — one that validates who you are and also projects an ideal version of yourself — can lift you up almost effortlessly over time." But it can also have dire consequences. Flora goes on to say, "In contrast, staying with the wrong crowd will leave you walking against the wind, having to exert more and more effort just to move forward."[11]

Becoming Part of a Group

Development and psychological maturation can lead to changes in our relationships to groups. We can have less of a need to be part of the "right crowd." We can become more comfortable being alone. But we can also develop a greater capacity to be part of a group. Erikson suggests that we become more comfortable in diverse groups as we begin to feel more secure and comfortable with who we are.

This is what happened for Annie, who talked about her "mommy friends," those relationships that develop with parents of your children's friends. Sometimes these connections are the result of structured parenting groups, sometimes they develop naturally with other women at the playground or in the neighborhood, and sometimes they are formed during school fundraisers. "When my first child was born, I didn't have time for anyone except my baby," Annie said. "Work was intense, and being a mom of a newborn was intense — I took only a six-week maternity leave. I barely had time for my husband, Jake, anymore. So I didn't make any mommy friends that time around. But besides that, I was sure that the nonworking parents would be critical of me for not being with my child all the time, and the professional moms would be critical of me for not working hard enough, or for having troubles balancing my work and personal life."

Annie was lonely even though she felt totally connected to and fulfilled by her new baby. Several years later, when her second child was born, Annie had a new attitude. "Something changed when my daughter Lily [her first] started preschool. I hadn't yet gotten pregnant with my second child, and I was sad about that. But I got involved in some activities at the school, and I started to have some — I don't know, I wouldn't have called them friends, but — acquaintances, I guess. The children started to have play dates, and Jake and I started doing things with a couple of the parents. Gradually, we became friendly with some of them, as couples. And we would do things together as families on weekends. I stopped feeling so lonely. It was kind of a big surprise."

What was even more surprising to Annie, as it is to many women, is that her friendships with the other mothers had a very different feel than any of her earlier relationships with women. "We haven't become best friends," she said. "We don't share all of our secrets. But there's a kind of comfort in knowing they're there. They've got my back, and I've got theirs."

Interestingly, some of these selections change over the course of our lifetimes, and of course with different life experiences. For instance, Sofia, whose friend Valeria brought her into a wonderful, supportive group, was surprised when Valeria began to be less accessible to her. "I thought I had done something wrong," Sofia said in her soft voice. "But then I found out that other women in the group were also feeling that way. We finally found out that Valeria was ill. She didn't want anyone to know about it. She kept it totally to herself. We weren't allowed to go with her to the doctor or even to bring her food, the way she would have done with any of us."

Sofia and her friends were puzzled by Valeria's attitude, until they realized that she was comfortable being the group leader, but not being intimate on a one-to-one basis with anyone. "I think she hated the idea of being dependent," said Sofia. Other women shared similar stories about important group members. "It's also a matter of gossip," said one divorcée who had been close friends with four other women for nearly thirty years. "You worry about what might be said behind your back. I live in a small town, and I ran into one of my friends when I was out on a date with a guy I was starting to like. I was terrified about the conversations that would go on behind my back."

Yet a number of the most active group members who talked with me said that there are "unspoken rules" about gossip. "You can try to understand something about one of the other women," said one member of a New York City mothers' group, "but you can't gossip. And it's totally not okay to share something that's told to you in confidence." She said, "It would be a stupid thing to do, actually, much as you might want to, because somebody will tell your friend, and they'll also say where they got the information, and then no one will ever tell you anything at all."

The Importance of Small Details

Harry Stack Sullivan, a famous American psychoanalyst, believed that psychological understanding and change come not from embracing psychological theory, but from paying attention to the tiny details of everyday life. That women grasp this concept intuitively is evident almost any time a group of women gets together. Intellectual matters may be discussed, feelings will be considered and explored, but inevitably someone will start to talk about some of the minutiae that Sullivan believed are the essence of life.

After her friend turned into a Bridezilla in the months leading up to her own wedding, twenty-seven-year-old Violet was determined to behave differently. Her experience is an echo of Sullivan's ideas. "When I was planning my own wedding," she said, "I tried not to be totally self-centered. But my friends were willing to listen while I obsessed about big and little things, from where to seat my grandma to what color the men's boutonnieres should be. My fiancé was excited that we were going to be married, and he wanted it to be a fun wedding. But he wasn't interested in all of the nitty-gritty. My girlfriends were genuinely interested." Women often appreciate the small, seemingly insignificant details of one another's lives.

What You Can Do

WHEN YOU WANT TO JOIN A GROUP

If you feel that you are being excluded from a group, make sure you are reading the situation correctly. Convinced that all of the other mothers were critical of her, Annie assumed that she could never belong to any of their groups. But once she started joining activities and got to know these mothers, she found that they had many things in common — including, she laughingly told me, a fear of being criticized and left out by the other parents.

Take a chance. Sometimes group members read the very things you do to protect yourself — keeping a distance, not appearing too interested — to mean that you do not want to join them. They might be just as anxious about being rejected by you as you are by them. Sure, that is not always the case, but how much can it hurt to take a chance?

If you do take that chance, and you are rejected, consider that not everyone in the group has rejected you. Try singling out one woman to say hello to every day. Annie discovered that one of the other mothers, who she thought was part of the "in-group," also felt left out. "And she was a really nice, smart, and interesting woman," Annie told me.

And finally, when nothing else works, let it go. Holding on to hurt and pain doesn't do you any good. If you cannot be part of an existing group, think about joining a different group or forming one of your own. You might also consider the advice of one active, outgoing sixty-six-year-old, who told me, "One day I realized that all of my friends had moved away or moved on, and I was alone with just my husband — whom I do love, but who isn't enough! So I started making a list of the women I knew who I might want to spend a little time with. I invited all of them to a meeting at my house to see who might be interested in joining me in a project I'd been thinking about for a while, but hadn't been able to get off the ground. We got together to talk about how we could provide diapers for families who couldn't afford to buy them; and when we'd finished coming up with ideas and plans, none of us wanted to go home. We spent six hours together that day. And now we meet once a month. We discuss business — we have a flourishing program now! And then we hang out and eat and visit."

You do not have to be part of a squad to have a valuable and meaningful friendship experience. You might join an organization that provides a service to those in need, or consider taking a class in something that interests you. Look at groups that you already belong to, as well. Salma's friends decided to add some structure to their long-standing group in order to "stretch their brains." In these ways you might very well find yourself feeling more connected to others and happier.

WHEN YOU ARE ALREADY IN A GROUP

When she returned to China, Alexandra said, she found herself making an extra effort to welcome outsiders into her group of friends. "I realized how hard it was to break into a group, and I knew from my own experience how lonely that can make you feel." She also realized that she was part of a much larger group than she had ever recognized before. "Some of my friends are more in the center of the group and some are more on the outside. But we are good friends, and we are a good, supportive group. A lot of us went to school together, so we have been friends for a long time. But now we have brought in other people — work friends, and now our boyfriends and husbands. We like doing things together."

Remember also that there needs to be room in a group for differences. One travel agent in her thirties told me that she had been part of a close-knit group since college. This group had expanded over the course of the years to include a wide range of friends, spouses, and now even some children. When I asked if she could tell me what had made the group last so long, she said, "I think part of the reason is that we all like each other. But we also allow for different interests and styles. Some of us like going to concerts, and some of us like going to the movies. And all of us like to eat! So sometimes we'll have a big dinner party, and we'll all bring food and wine and we'll spend hours together, talking, singing, eating... but sometimes we'll break off into smaller groups, doing the different things we like to do. We don't feel like we all have to do the same thing."

Mary, whose friends supported her through the loss of her husband, said, "You know, I'm very close to the women in my Bible study group. My church is very, very important to me. But the funny thing is, we don't all believe the same thing. Sometimes we talk about who God is, and we've found that none of us seems to have the same God. He's different for each one of us. And that works fine. We have similar beliefs, and mostly similar values. So if we have differences in this, even though it's a very important part of our connection to each other, it's okay. Maybe it even makes it a little better to have some differences."

As we have seen, being part of an admired clique can also have lasting fallout. There is a price to be paid for being part of the "in-group," such as losing your independence or sense of individuality.

Psychoanalysts, group therapists, and many others agree that making space for differences is crucial to human connectedness in general and to healthy friendships in particular. At the same time, they tell us that one of the most important ways to undo prejudice and exclusion, and the hurt and anger that inevitably follow, is to recognize the humanness of people who are not part of your particular group. Naomi Novik's fairy tale beautifully captures this lesson, ending with the heroine, Agnieszka, understanding something of her mortal enemy's humanity. Agnieszka says, "We looked at one

• another. For a moment, through the winding smoke between us, I might have been the daughter she'd hoped for. She might have been my teacher and my guide. We might never have been enemies at all."[12]

Although it is unlikely that making space for both connection and difference will take away all prejudice, hatred, and resentment, accepting and even embracing dissimilarity can improve your ability to feel good in and out of group situations. Knowing that we and our very closest friends can have disparate perspectives and that we and our sworn enemies can have much in common can be puzzling and upsetting. Such awareness can shake up a tightly bound group that values commonality. But in the end, embracing differences expand your self-knowledge and sense of well-being. It will deepen some of your friendships, sometimes in surprising ways. If you are not a group person, it might actually make you feel more comfortable the next time you are in a group situation. And it will make it easier to turn your back on any group that does not want you as a member.

6

*How Many Friends
Do You Need?*

'M LEARNING SOMETHING NEW ABOUT FRIENDSHIP these days," said Daphne, who divorced her husband and ended her relationship with her best friend after finding them in bed together. "I used to have a bunch of women who I thought were friends, but I think the truth was, I didn't really know what friendship meant. Some of them deserted me during the divorce. They weren't willing, or able, to be there for me during the hardest time of my life." Always a caregiver, Daphne discovered that when she needed care herself, the number of women she could count on quickly diminished. "I was really vulnerable during the early days of the separation and divorce. I lost the two people I trusted most in the world — my husband and my best friend. And I discovered that lots of the women I had thought liked me only wanted me to take care of them."

Daphne's caregiving nature had always been what connected her to many of the women in her life. "Even though I look like an outgoing person, I'm actually shy. But I can open up when someone needs me. As my friends disappeared, and I thought about starting to make new ones, I decided that I would be much more discriminating about who I would let myself get close to. But it's not so easy to make new friends at my age. What are you going to do, just say to someone, 'Hey, I kind of like you. Will you be my friend — but first will you let me know if you're willing to make this a mutually supportive relationship?' I spend a lot more time with my kids and my family now, and a fair amount of time on my own. I've accepted that making new friends will be slow. That's actually a good thing. I'll make sure that I know someone really well before I trust her — or him — completely. But I can't help but feel bad sometimes, like when I look at the Facebook pages of some of the women I used to spend time with. They have so many friends. I have some, but not many, and right now nobody I'm really close to."

I have met women of all different ages and experiences who worry about not having enough friends. An outgoing waitress with a gold tooth that flashed when she smiled said, "When I was little, every time I saw my grandmother, she would ask me how many friends I had. I was always ashamed to admit that I only had one best friend. As I got older, her words echoed in my brain. I have a lot of friends now, but I wonder if it would be enough for Gramma; and I also wonder why it was so important to her."

Why does anyone count the number of friends she has? Of course, one modern reason is social media, where friends and followers, likes and shares are visible to us and anyone else who happens to take a look. When the poet Alex Morritt asked in his book *Impromptu Scribe,* "How can anyone truly claim to have eleven hundred friends?" he was of course pointing out the oddness of the very concept of "friend" these days.[1] The term, once reserved for people you know and like, is used now to describe someone you may never have met in person, who might be vaguely connected to someone else you know, who likes something you've posted on social media.

The question of how many friends we need, however, is one that troubles many of the women I interviewed. An office manager in her forties told me that she has many acquaintances, "but only three women who I would actually call friends. I wish I could be one of those women with a large group of girlfriends who meet up for a glass of wine or a cup of tea and go away for girls' weekends, but that's never been me. I just don't open up like that."

A travel agent who has a large network of women and men she calls her "dearest friends" said that she could not imagine a life without them. "I feel sorry for women who don't have a bunch of friends. They must be so sad." There is a belief that the more friends you have, the happier you are, but is that an accurate perception? It turns out that the number of friends is less important than the role they play in your life.

Research has found that friendships support mental and physical health in a variety of ways.[2] We know, even without the research confirming it, that friends help us process emotions, but in many cases they also help us stay physically healthy. One study found that a lack of social connection was worse for physical well-being than smoking, obesity, or high blood pressure.[3] The connection is not magical. Social support can help us manage stress, which can reduce the impact of stress hormones, high blood pressure, and other potential physical damage. Friends can also push us to exercise and socialize, which can directly affect our health.[4] Of course, they can influence us to behave in ways that are bad for our health too, especially in adolescence, when we may be all too ready to succumb to peer pressure to eat, drink, and party too much.

Many women talked about walking, jogging, or going to the gym with friends. Others said that they had found it helpful to diet with a group. As one new mother put it, "I can't get this baby fat off by myself. I have three friends who are all working to get back in shape after a pregnancy. We support, encourage, and push each other. It's a great system. I don't feel all alone, and I don't feel bad about myself when I go off track. I just call one of my friends and get a pep talk to get started again. It helps knowing that every one of us is in the same boat!"

Graciela, a translator with long, dark curls, told me that she was a recovering alcoholic. "I'm thirty-five and single. All of my old friends are married and have children. That's what they focus on. I feel like an outsider, a weirdo. I love to see them, of course, and their babies and children, but I'm not so interested in what they want to talk about. I mean, it's lovely, but it's not what I'm thinking about or doing. I feel like a freak around them. I have a rich and fulfilling life, but it's hard to make friends.

"I don't go out drinking anymore, which was the way I used to socialize. So a lot of my friends come from Alcoholics Anonymous. We go to the movies together, or out for a cup of coffee after a meeting. When I'm really lonely, that's when I could see myself having a drink. So instead, I call my sponsor or another AA buddy, or I go to a meeting. They help me stay on track and off the bottle."

Sometimes the influence is less direct. Femi, an architect in her thirties, talked about an older friend who kept smoking cigarettes next to her while she was pregnant. "I said I wasn't comfortable with her smoking around me, and she apologized and said she would stop. I know she tried, but she just couldn't help it. She would light up automatically. I didn't want to keep asking her not to do it, so I would get up and go out of the room when she pulled out a cigarette. I didn't see her for a little while near the end of my pregnancy, but I didn't think a whole lot about it, since I was super-busy and there had always been times when we didn't get together so much.

But right after the baby was born, she came to visit and told me that she had stopped smoking, and that it was because of me.

"She was so ashamed that I had had to leave the room and that she couldn't stop herself from having a cigarette, even though she loved me and didn't want to hurt my baby, that she went for help. I was sorry that she was embarrassed, but glad that she's stopped smoking. And I can see how much healthier she is already, so I don't feel too bad about it. In a roundabout way, I helped her get healthier."

The Numbers Game

Two questions emerge, both from this research and from women like the waitress whose Gramma wanted a friend count. First, how many friends do we need in order to reap these emotional and physical health benefits? And second, how close does a friend need to be in order to make a difference?

The answers to these questions might surprise you. A number of studies have shown that the advantages of friendship are available whether you have a network of three or three hundred; and furthermore, that so-called superficial links can provide many of the same outcomes as more intense bonds. Women told me of one special friendship that has lasted for decades, although they seldom actually saw each other in person. "But when we do," said one writer, echoing the words of many, "it's like we have never been apart." People noted this about the American author Edith Wharton: "Her friends are few but of long standing."[5]

An airline attendant in her forties told me, "I grew up with the television show *Friends*. There were six young adults who helped each other manage all of the ups and downs, bumps and glitches that came along as they tried to figure out how to become grown-ups. Sure, they were silly and naive and sometimes downright stupid, but they cared about each other and went to bat for each other. I wish I had just one friend like that." She went on to say that, on the other hand, she was proud of her independence. "I think some women get lost in this idea that we need to be close to lots of other women. Of course," she adds, "I didn't grow up in the era of Facebook, when you can see how many friends other girls have, and you feel bad and ashamed that you aren't participating in all of the so-called fun."

Bridget, a thirty-six-year-old writer, told me that she was more comfortable on her own than with a lot of other people. "I'm not socially isolated, but I don't need lots of friends," she said. "It almost doesn't compute for me when people talk about those crazy Facebook numbers. I've got two really good friends, and that's plenty." In her book *Quiet,* the author Susan Cain writes that this preference for "less stimulation, as when they sip wine with a close friend, solve a crossword puzzle, or read a book," can be a sign that you are an introvert, a quality frequently undervalued in contemporary society. Although extroverts get more attention, she writes, there are many great people, including Rosa Parks and Eleanor Roosevelt, who had an impact on the world not in spite of, but because they were introverts.[6]

Research tells us that the number of friends we have diminishes naturally over time.[7] This diminution is a normal part of the process of moving from late adolescence into early adulthood. Sometimes it happens quietly, as we change our focus and our goals, and sometimes the shift is painful. Sue, a fifty-seven-year-old interior designer, told me, "I was so busy, putting all of my attention into my family and my career. And then, when everything was going smoothly in that part of my life, I looked around and realized I used to have so many more friends than I do now. What happened to them all?"

Interestingly, a report in *Live Science* tells us that, at least in the

United States, there is a general decrease in the number of people we consider to be friends. According to one study, in 1985 Americans reported an average of about three (2.95, to be exact) friends whom they could talk to about important issues. By 2004 that number had fallen to an average of about two (2.04).[8] And this despite the advent of friend counts in the hundreds and even thousands on social media. It appears that we are struggling with social isolation and loneliness in the midst of a sea of so-called friendships. Yet many women told me that they stay in touch with friends through social media. "It's my lifeline," said one busy professional. "I get to chat and connect every day with friends who I don't see for months at a time. I don't think I could handle my life without it!" Social media can, however, also add to the sense that you are being left out of something important. Whether it is the number of friends you do or don't have, or the activities you are or are not participating in, the ability to see what other folks are doing has created a numbers anxiety of its own. A fear of being left out is so much a part of today's culture that it has its own acronym: FOMO, fear of missing out.

The *New York Times* writer Jenna Wortham describes this contemporary dilemma[9] beautifully. She writes that she was settling in to enjoy a quiet night at home, when "my iPhone began flashing with notifications from a handful of social networking sites, each a beacon of information about what my friends were doing." Whether they were eating at trendy restaurants, drinking milkshakes together, or going to a movie, they appeared to be having so much fun that Wortham felt restless and uneasy. Her peaceful, solitary evening had lost its appeal.

She was struggling with FOMO. This anxiety arises when you don't go to a party or some other social event, and fear you'll miss out on something really important. The British newspaper columnist Rosie Boycott calls it a "thoroughly modern malaise."[10] A recent college grad told me, "When I was in college, it was an easy thing to just go out and run into friends. But sometimes I wanted to stay home and wash my hair, give myself a manicure, and hang out in my sweats and read or watch a movie. It was hard to do that then, and it's hard to do it now, because I'm always worried that I'll find out I missed out on something important."

A radiologist in her thirties said, "I'm not much of a party person. I had an eating disorder during most of my adolescence and through my twenties. When I was anorexic, I wouldn't go out because I didn't want to be uncomfortable about my eating. People were always looking to see how much I actually ate. Then I started bingeing and purging, and I didn't want people to see me gorge myself and didn't want them to think I was throwing up — which I was.

"I'm shy," she told me, "and it's hard for me to socialize. The eating disorder gave me an excuse for staying home. I'd rather stay home now too. But now I get lonely. And it's hard to go out. I prefer to be home with my family than out with a bunch of friends who are drinking and eating too much in order to have a good time. Every year the hospital throws a big Christmas party, and I always feel torn. I want to celebrate with my friends at work because it's the end of the really difficult season, and we're all exhausted and deserve to have some fun together; but I don't really find being at a party, even with my good friends, to be that much fun. The one time I didn't go, though, I felt miserable. I was sure I was missing out on something really important."

An IT specialist said something similar, echoing the words of many. "I'm not a big drinker, but my office has happy hour every Thursday after work. I like hanging out with my work friends, and I don't want to look like a party pooper or anything; but I'd really rather go out with a couple of them at a time, so that we can actually talk about things that matter. But that's not how it works, and if I don't go to happy hour, I could miss out on something significant." When I asked what that something might be, she said, "You never know. It might be social, like that a work friend is engaged or pregnant, or work-related, like someone has been let go or is leaving because they have new job. If I don't go, I'll be the last one to find out, and that's embarrassing."

For many women, social media is often both a cause of and a solution to FOMO. On the one hand, seeing pictures of friends having a grand time without you can contribute to feelings of loneliness and lower self-esteem. On the other hand, social media provides a tool for contact and connection with other women who have as little time as you do. The weary mother with three small children told me that the Internet was her lifeline. Like many other busy women, she belonged to several online mothers' groups. "It's where I go when I need someone to figuratively hold my hand while my child is going through the terrible twos, or when I need advice about almost anything. I can also sell my kids' outgrown clothes and toys and buy used ones from other mothers. These are my friends, even though I have never met most of them in person."

Friends, as we have seen, give us a sense of normalcy. Through words and actions, they let us know that we are okay, even when we have doubts about ourselves. Sometimes just seeing or reading about other women who are going through some of the same things we are struggling with can make us feel more comfortable with our own difficulties. Whether on the Internet or in person, a larger friend group can supply a wider range of possible mirrors, making it more likely that you will find someone who knows how you feel because she has been there herself. This is how it was for Marie Hélène, who, now in her forties, belonged to a large group of women friends that had started in college. "My best friend brought me into the group," she told me. "And that's how it went. Someone else's best friend would bring in a new girl, and we just kept growing." Like many such groups, this one had an informal leader, Cécile, a charismatic woman who often initiated get-togethers and activities for the entire group. "She's a ball of energy," Marie Hélène said.

"Sometimes I felt sad," she went on, "because Cécile did not seem to like me quite as much as she liked some of the other women in the group. I thought it was because I was different somehow, maybe not as outgoing as she was, or because I was working and started a family before most of the other women in the group. But there was one other woman who was part of the group and who was like me, having children and working too. We would talk sometimes, and I confessed my insecurities about Cécile. My friend said she'd gone through the same thing with Cécile, until she realized that she — Cécile — was not able to be close friends with anyone, but that she needed people to admire her and look up to her all the time. She thought that Cécile might be having a hard time with us because we were more serious and because we had a life outside the group. It made me feel so much better. I was able to let go of worrying about whether or not Cécile liked me and just enjoy the times I was with the group."

Changes over Time

Like some of the women I talked with, you may not notice right away that you have fewer friends than you used to. Or, like others, you may observe and mourn the loss of those old companions. The beloved author Nora Ephron said, "The thing with friends when you get older is they can't be replaced. When you're thirty, you accumulate friends and you shed friends and you get closer at certain moments to some than others. And you have a huge bench of friends. And then that's just not true."

One source of pain can come from trying to hold on to old friends who are no longer available. This is what happened to another recent college grad who told me that she loved her sorority sisters more than anyone else in the world. "We just don't hang out together anymore," she said. "We all have busy lives, and of course some of us don't even live in the same town. I try to make it my business to see everyone as often as I can, and I try to get the whole group together regularly. It just makes me so sad to think that we won't ever have the same kind of connection that we used to have. I don't want to let that happen. Ever."

Other women were more accepting of the natural progression and change. "My life has changed, and so of course the women I'm friends with have changed too," said a working mother in her forties. In their book *Between Women,* Luise Eichenbaum and Susie Orbach write, "The stresses and strains of managing work, partners, children, and friends is very real."[11] These authors remind us that the quality of our relationships is as important as the quantity. Studies in social science back up this belief, although in one series of studies a group of researchers found that there is a difference between age groups in this regard. In a thirty-year longitudinal study, they found that the quantity of friendships a person has in her twenties can be an indicator of the quality of friendships she will have in her fifties. On the other hand, they found that the quality, not the quantity, of these social connections in our thirties was the better predictor for healthy connections in our fifties.[12]

Other research has shown that deeply intense friendships are not necessarily more important than regular, comfortable contact with someone whom you consider a casual acquaintance. Paula Hawkins, who wrote the best-selling thriller *The Girl on the Train,* says friendships between women are not all the same. "The troubled relationship I had with my best friend in my twenties is by no means representative of all my friendships. Some are sunnier, they've been smoother sailing — even if I sometimes wonder if that is because the waters are shallower."[13]

A number of studies found that seeing one another within the context of familiar albeit not necessarily intense or deeply meaningful activities can be an important part of a healthy, supportive network.[14] Occasionally going out for coffee with a woman you see at your weekly yoga class, or for a walk with a neighbor, may be enough for such a connection. Other kinds of networks can also provide support, as Graciela, the translator who is an alcoholic in recovery, explained. Structured support groups, religious organizations, business associations, and political parties can provide comfort and connection.

These contacts do not have to occur in a structured setting, however. Links may form spontaneously or around a specific activity. A single woman in her late fifties told me that she had three traveling buddies. "We get together to talk about our next trip or to go over things from the last one. We don't have a lot in common other than a shared love of travel, but that's enough. It keeps us all centered." And a divorced lab technician with grown children said, "I have one friend who's my 'movie companion.' We don't even like the same movies, but we go to all of the new releases together, so we see each other a couple of times a month. It's a steady, comfortable connection. We have dinner, catch up on each other's lives, and talk about the movie we just saw. And then we go home and don't talk till we make arrangements for our next movie night."

Numerous women told me that as they got older, they were more involved in groups where the women had little in common except a particular interest — for example, reading, going to the theater or concerts, political activism, memoir-writing, crafts, or even simply shopping. Juliana, who learned to be close to women only in adulthood, created and ran a charitable organization with a group of friends. A fifty-seven-year-old retiree organized a group to read in the local Head Start program. The group expanded to do other volunteer service. "We didn't know each other before we started this activity," this woman told me. "And I'm not sure that we would have become friends even if we had met socially. But the bond of doing an important service can't be described. We consider ourselves close friends, even though we meet only once a month."

Paula Hawkins writes, "There are few truly good things about getting older, but here, in my opinion, are two. First, no one bothers to catcall you in the street any longer. And second, friendship gets easier."[15]

One of the reasons that senior communities and assisted living residences work for many women is that they have both autonomy and connection at a time when they can no longer live on their own. An eighty-nine-year-old widow who was confined to a wheelchair told me that she would never have been friends with most of the other women in her assisted living facility, "but I like having my regular lunch and dinner companions. I'm very lucky, because my kids and grandkids come to visit me all the time. But some of the other folks here aren't so lucky, and the residents and staff are the only people they see.

"But even for me, it's nice to know that I'm going to have someone to talk to during my meals. I'm not in great shape, so I couldn't get out when I was living alone, and my friends aren't in good shape either — if they're even still alive. So I'm friends with the folks I see here, even if I wouldn't have been when I was younger." She chuckled and added, "You know that old song that goes 'If you can't be with the one you love, love the one you're with'? That's how it is with these friends. We talk about our children and grandchildren, and our life before we moved here. We have crazy-different backgrounds, families, and politics, which we don't talk about at all. But most of us don't remember what we told each other from day to day, so none of that's important. It's just nice to know that you're going to see a familiar face at lunch and dinner."

What You Can Do

According to evolutionary psychologists, we humans are social animals. We need companionship, but we need more than other warm bodies. One of the interesting findings of neuropsychiatry and psychoanalysis in recent years is that we have specific needs for connection. For one thing, we crave a sense that other people see us. Peter Fonagy, a leading figure in attachment theory, says that a child learns to know herself through seeing her reflection in the faces of her parents and caregivers.[16] Heinz Kohut, who developed the therapeutic approach called self psychology, says that "mirroring" is a prerequisite not only to healthy development, but also to emotional well-being, from birth to death.[17]

As we have seen, the number of friends you have is far less important, over time, than whether or not you feel seen and validated by the friends you do have. This can be many friends who know and reflect different parts of you, or one friend who knows you inside out and cares for you, flaws and all. The psychoanalyst Jessica Benjamin calls this our need for "recognition,"[18] which is not necessarily about showing off, but rather the need to know that someone whom we respect, admire, or simply feel close to really knows who we are and cares about us, even with our less-than-lovable flaws. This is, of course, a basic need. But research has shown us that we also simply need to be connected.

FOMO, then, may not reflect a fear of being left out, but rather a basic need for contact. You may feel worried about not being "in" or missing out on something important. But in truth, the underlying message you are receiving from your inner self is that you want to connect. This fear of not being connected is often the root of loneliness. The psychoanalyst Robert Stolorow[19] has written that when we don't feel connected, we feel that no one can understand us and, furthermore, that we are not part of the human race. This lack of connection, according to a number of studies, can cause loneliness, depression, and hopelessness.[20]

So how many friends do you really need? There is no magic number. Nor do your friendships need to be deep or intense. The goal is surprisingly simple: try to make and stay in some kind of contact with other people. Like the elderly woman in the wheelchair, you might just find someone nearby whom you can talk to every so often, even if that person does not share your values or your life experiences. You could join a walking group, even if you don't particularly like to walk. The benefit of being outside and getting a little exercise is enhanced by the fact that you are also spending a little time with potential friends. Or you might prefer to join a group of people who do share your interests. That's what happened with Daphne. She joined a local political group "because I wanted to take some kind of political action, but the extra benefit was that I felt connected to these other people who shared my values. I also reconnected to myself, to a part of myself that had been missing since I was in college and involved in all kinds of student action committees. And," she added slowly, "being with them gives me hope."

Maybe, then, this feeling of connection to someone else, and the resulting reconnection to parts of yourself, is the true key to women's friendships.

7

~

Should Friends Give Advice to Friends?

N THE COURSE OF A SINGLE WEEK, THREE WOMEN TOLD me about the hidden misery of being asked to be part of a friend's wedding party. Violet, the outgoing twenty-seven-year-old who was bridesmaid to her Bridezilla friend, has also been maid of honor and wedding guest more times than she liked to count. She said, "The first time a good friend gets engaged, you're so excited and pleased for her. And the first time someone asks you to be her maid of honor, you feel really special! It's such a compliment! And then you find out what's involved — that basically you're her servant from that moment till the day after her wedding. It's her day, and of course you're going to do what she wants. But what you don't expect is that she's going to want to run your life — that she is going to believe that just about everything you do that entire time should be under her control."

Thirty-four-year-old Sara said, "My best friend's wedding destroyed our relationship. I'd always laughed about the idea of a Bridezilla, but I hadn't seen one in action before. But she really did turn into a monster, without an ounce of consideration for anyone else. We had to buy expensive, unattractive dresses — well, that's standard — and spend money most of us didn't have on an all-out shower and a destination bachelorette party, and smile while we did it. There was no talking to her about other possibilities."

And forty-one-year-old Lisa said, "Don't let anyone tell you that only young, straight women go nuts over their wedding plans. I didn't think we were going to get my best friend and her future wife down the aisle, because they obsessed endlessly over every detail. I worried that all their friends were going to be so frustrated with their perfectionism that they'd end up without anybody at the wedding!"

The web is full of advice for women whose BFFs have turned into Bridezillas. There's even a popular, long-running TV series about the phenomenon. But when it's happening to you, it can turn from a joke to a nightmare.

Of course, brides aren't the only ones who can take the need to control a friend to an extreme. It can happen at any age and any stage of life. Juliana, now in her fifties, who was sent as a little girl from her native Vietnam to boarding school in England, told me, "My best friend was Mila, another girl from my country. She was a year older than I and had been at the school a year longer. So she took me under her wing, even calling me her little sister." At first Juliana felt comforted and safe with her new friend's attention. But soon she discovered that there was a painful price to this sense of security. "She couldn't bear it if I did anything even slightly different from her," Juliana said. "We all wore the same school uniform, so there wasn't an issue about dress. But if I wanted to eat a piece of fruit that she didn't like, that wasn't okay. If I talked to a girl who didn't have her stamp of approval, she became mean and nasty to me."

A thirty-five-year-old working mother said, "I had a good friend who decided that I wasn't raising my children correctly. She was always, always telling me what I should and shouldn't do with them, from what my highly allergic little girl should eat to what time my kids should go to bed. It was like a bad mother-in-law joke, only worse." A forty-year-old single professional spoke of a former best friend who "seemed to think that she had the right to tell me what guys I could date and when I needed to get out of a relationship." And a fifty-five-year-old executive assistant said, "I have a sort-of friend at work who's always telling me what I should wear and how I should fix my hair. The other day, after I got my hair cut a little shorter than usual, everybody was telling me how great I looked. But this woman looked at me and said, 'You got your hair cut. I liked it better the other way.' Maybe I should be grateful for her honesty, but the truth is, I don't think it's really about whether or not the haircut looks good. I think she just likes to boss me around."

What makes women friends think they have the right to tell us what to do?

Bossy Friends Come in Many Forms

Before answering that question, perhaps we should ask if calling someone "bossy" is just a way of criticizing strong women. "I want every little girl who someone says 'they're bossy' to be told instead, 'you have leadership skills,'" says a widespread Facebook post from Sheryl Sandberg, author of *Lean In: Women, Work, and the Will to Lead,* the popular but controversial book about women in the business world.[1] Of course no one likes to be called bossy. But as one blogger responded, "Bossy is not leadership. In fact, bossy is the opposite of leadership. Being bossy is a skill that every two-year-old has mastered. Bossy is 'shut up and do it my way; I know best!' Leadership is the opposite."[2] Yet Sandberg points out that some behavior that is labeled bossy in women is accepted and even celebrated in men. And when you think about it, how often is a man described as bossy?

Calling a woman bossy is probably a criticism some of the time, but not always. Many of the women I spoke with said that they saw a very definite difference between bossiness and leadership. Juliana echoed the blogger: "A bossy woman is hard to be friends with, because she always thinks she is right. A good leader knows how to listen — to her staff, her followers, her leaders, or her colleagues. And a good friend knows how to listen to her friends," she said. "A bossy woman is not that far from being a bully."

Juliana, now an activist who works to help women around the world find ways to move out of poverty and enslavement, believes that women become bossy friends when they feel that their own lives are not in their control. "Show me a controlling or bullying female," she told me, "and I'll show you someone who feels insecure and unsupported in her life."

Not everyone agrees. Violet told me that her bossy girlfriend had grown up feeling entitled. "She's the only girl in a family of four children. Her brothers and her parents all spoil her to death. She has never been asked to think about anyone but herself. The funny thing is, despite being pampered and indulged, she was always a good friend until she started with the wedding stuff. But when I thought back about it, after the fact, I realized that what I'd liked about her was her sense of fun and adventure. I'm kind of quiet and not so adventurous myself, so I always let her take the lead. I felt safe doing stuff with her because she was so sure of herself. But when she started planning her wedding, I realized that her self-confidence had to do with her sense that she's always right and that therefore her needs should always come first."

The feeling that you are always right is often related to a failure of empathy. A friend not strong on empathy may not have the ability to experience an internal version of what other people are thinking or feeling. Although she thinks she knows what is right for everyone else, she may often miss the mark because she does not really understand her friends' feelings and needs. A combined lack of empathy and sense of always being right might be a sign of narcissism. This now-popular term is often used to mean self-centered to the point of harming others who do not meet our needs. Psychoanalysts view narcissism as a self-centeredness that is not necessarily intentionally cruel, although it can result in hurtful actions. Most narcissists have difficulty recognizing differences between their own needs and those of others, thus leading them to meet their own desires even when it causes pain to someone else. Undine Spragg, the heroine of Edith Wharton's novel *The Custom of the Country,* is a great example of this kind of friend. Anything she does or says to anyone else is always in the service of her own needs. She wants her friends to be happy because when people around her are content, she feels good. In fact, Wharton tells us, Undine "wanted to make everybody about her happy. If only everyone would do as she wished she would never be unreasonable."[3]

But not all bossy friends are narcissists — some tell other people what they should do because they genuinely think those people will be happier as a result.

Liz and Eileen, the teens who were "perfectly matched" in high school, became close again after college. "Well, we didn't really have a choice," Liz said, with her contagious smile. "Eileen married my older brother." Now in their late thirties, they agree that their relationship can be difficult at times. "One of the big problems is that Eileen says I'm too bossy," Liz told me. "I think it's because I have very definite opinions, and I don't have any hesitation about sharing them with her. And she doesn't always like them." Eileen said, "There's no arguing with Liz. It's her way or the highway."

A case in point occurred when Eileen was trying to decide whether or not to send her eight-year-old son to camp. "I thought it was a terrible idea," Liz said. "And I told her so. He's too young. Why does he need to go away? What purpose does it serve?" Eileen said, "I told her that my son was the one who brought it up. One of his friends was going, and he wanted to go as well. I went to camp when I was eight. It was a wonderful experience! I wanted my son to have the same opportunity." None of her arguments changed Liz's opinion. "It's hard for us to agree to disagree," Eileen said.

"We don't either of us like to lose," Liz added.

Making Room for Difference

Taylor Swift and her #SquadGoals friends elicit conflicting feelings about a leader who sets a standard for her best friends. On the one hand, as one Internet post puts it, "It's so inspiring how Taylor Swift makes it clear that you can achieve your wildest dreams when you believe in yourself."[4] The squad seems to be an integral part of Swift's self-confidence and to elevate her friends almost to her status. As Lindsay Putnam writes in the *New York Post,* Swift and her squad have become the "gold standard for anyone seeking a close-knit yet undeniably fabulous group of friends."[5]

Yet can any group of women look and act so much like one another without some loss of individuality? Commenters, from Amy Zimmerman in the *Daily Beast*[6] to the British fashion legend Naomi Campbell,[7] suggest that there may not be much room for women who are part of this elite group to express their differences. In the film *Clueless,* the classic backhanded feminist romp loosely based on Jane Austen's *Emma,* Cher Horowitz's friend Tai is so drawn in by Cher that she seems to lose her own identity. This is another example of "gilt by association," of course. Tai gives up who she is so that she can be connected to and get some borrowed social status and "glitter" from a friend she admires.

Even as a child Juliana was unwilling to give up her own personality to her friend. She told me that she decided it was better to have no friends at all than to have to submit to the control of someone like her schoolmate Mila. So she quietly pulled away, using her studies as an excuse. "I just always had some reading to do, or a lesson to work on, or I needed to go to the library." She even took to reading a book during meals instead of chatting with Mila as she had been doing previously. Eventually Mila stopped trying to engage with her, although, Juliana said, "I don't think she ever forgave me. But I couldn't have a sense of who I was with her. She couldn't tolerate my being my own person." Juliana feared that all friendships would require the same sacrifice, so she spent the rest of her school life isolating herself from other girls.

Should a Friend Tell a Friend . . . ?

Nicole, a forty-one-year-old banker, said, "I used to think you could and should tell a good friend what you think. But I learned the hard way to keep my mouth shut. My best friend and her husband had a terrible relationship. She was always complaining about how unkind and critical he was. He never said anything nice to her, told her she was looking old and fat, and had an affair with another friend of ours. Finally, she packed up and left him and moved back in with her parents. All of her friends were so relieved that she finally stood up to him, and we all supported her in every way we could. I think they even started divorce proceedings, but then a few months later he begged her to give him a second chance, and she fell for it.

"I was worried about her, so I told her that I didn't think it was a good idea. I said that he wasn't trustworthy, but she didn't listen. And after that she stopped talking to me. No big blowup or anything like that. She just was always too busy to hang out, or to get coffee, or even to talk on the phone. I got the message. I stopped trying. It makes me sad, but I guess she felt I would have been a better friend if I'd just sucked it up, kept my opinions to myself, and was there to support her. And maybe she's right. If I had it to do over again, maybe I'd do it differently."

Nicole was not motivated by sheer bossiness, and she was describing a dilemma many women face. Do you tell a friend when you think she is making a mistake with a romantic relationship, or do you keep your mouth shut and support her, no matter what? How do you define yourself as a friend in this kind of situation?

Some women told me that they would give their honest opinion no matter what the consequences. Others said that they would give it only if asked, or if they thought their friend or her children were in danger. But almost everyone told me they felt it was a "no win" situation. "If you say something, you take the risk of losing your friend," Nicole said. "But if you don't say something, you feel like you're not being a good friend."

Complicating the picture even more, sometimes not saying something can damage a friendship as badly as speaking up. "Friends are supposed to tell you the truth, even if it hurts, and even if you get mad at them," said one woman in her thirties, still in pain from discovering that her husband had been unfaithful and that her friends had known about it and never said anything to her. That this issue is such a popular topic for books, movies, and television speaks to how often it must occur. But as one of these movie titles puts it, *It's Complicated*. Women do take their cheating spouses back, and in the process they may reject the very friends who supported them in the days after they discovered the infidelity, when they were hurt and hostile toward their partner. In my work I have seen a number of different reasons for such rejections, including embarrassment or a desire to bury the hatchet with a spouse without being reminded of past problems by a friend. Sometimes, in a psychological maneuver called projection, you can be unfairly blamed for the difficulties with which you sympathized. This is what happened with Nicole, whose friend stayed with her husband and ended their friendship.

In the popular novel *Big Little Lies,* Liane Moriarty opens up the question of how much you can — and should — do when a woman you care about is in an abusive relationship. The question is not an easy one to answer at the best of times. On the one hand, it is hard to assess what is actually going on in anyone else's relationship, for several reasons. What looks untenable to us may be totally normal to someone else. Also, as is true for Moriarty's character Celeste, many women feel the need to keep their hurt to themselves. Celeste "pretended so very hard for so very long and there was nobody here except the two of them," Moriarty writes.[8] Upsetting that kind of an applecart can be serious business for a friendship. On the other hand, none of us wants to sit by while a friend is physically or emotionally mistreated, and we certainly do not want to ignore the potential that real harm could come to her.

A similar question comes up over and over again in my practice: What do you do when you suspect a friend has an eating disorder? Do you confront her, offer support, make suggestions, arrange an intervention? Or does a good friend ignore the evidence and assume that when she's ready, she'll get help? The questions are the same concerning a friend who drinks too much. Bholale, a dark-eyed forty-nine-year-old who works as a paralegal, told me about a longtime friend who was getting drunk on a regular basis. "I tried to say something, but she didn't listen. So one day I asked her husband if he would talk to her about it. He said, 'When she's ready, she'll do something about it.' And he was right. I don't know if he ever talked to her about our conversation. But when she was ready, she got help and stopped drinking."

It is not always easy to know when to offer advice, when to make an active intervention, when to keep your opinions to yourself and simply offer support and comfort. Or when to simply give up — a solution that could mean leaving a friendship altogether. But almost any expression of your own thoughts about what a friend is doing — or not doing — to her body can lead to trouble. Jacey, a twenty-three-year-old graduate student, worried that her friend Lese was bingeing and purging. "She was the life of the party, would drink and eat a ton when we were out with our friends, and then she'd disappear into the bathroom for forty-five minutes. We had roomed together in college, so I knew she used to throw up. I would smell it in the bathroom. But I thought she had stopped. When I finally said something to her, she told me to butt out. I told her I was only speaking up because I loved her and was worried about her. But she wouldn't talk about it with me at all. I don't know what happened, because it got too uncomfortable for me to be around her. I started to make some new friends at work, and I didn't hang out with the same crowd anymore. I just couldn't watch Lese do what she was doing. It felt so . . . dishonest."

The same can happen when a friend has either gained or lost a lot of weight. We all know how delicate an issue it can be to discuss a friend's weight with her, and most of us avoid saying anything that could possibly be hurtful about body size, diet, or appearance. But some women believe that expressing their opinion will make a difference. An actress who was struggling to lose the pounds she had put on during a pregnancy told me that one friend "simply looked me up and down and said, 'You've got to do something about that weight.' As if I didn't think about it 24/7. I was so hurt and so angry, I didn't talk to her again for weeks."

Aurora, a fifty-three-year-old middle school teacher who was still grieving her mother's death, was wearing a lavender hijab when we met. She said that she had once told her best friend that she was afraid the friend had taken her dieting too far. "She had lost so much weight that she looked like a prisoner of war," Aurora said. "I told her that I was worried about her health and about her children, since she couldn't be setting a very good example for them of how to eat. But she got furious with me. She told me I was hurting her feelings, that she knew it was because I was jealous that she had gotten so thin, and that I just wanted to destroy her happiness. I tried to explain that she was right, I was jealous at first, when she lost the weight and was looking so svelte, but that now I was just worried about her. And that even when I was jealous, I didn't want to destroy her happiness. I said I wasn't that kind of person, and that if she thought I was, she had not been the friend I thought she was. Things went downhill from there."

These problems can also occur when a friend is struggling with drugs or dangerous sexual behavior. When friends try to intervene, they are often met with hostility and resistance.

Yet some women complain about the opposite: friends who do not say anything.

Yolanda, a single woman in her late fifties, told me that she had struggled with alcoholism and an eating disorder throughout her adolescence. "I gained a lot of weight when I was twelve or thirteen, and then I started drinking heavily. I thought the alcohol helped curb my appetite, and for a while it did. I lost a lot of weight on my alcohol-only diet. But then I started eating again. I wish my friends had stepped in. They should have stood up to me. Sure, I would have been angry, and maybe my feelings would have been hurt. But a good friend will put up with that in order to help out. I would have been grateful after a while."

I heard such comments from many women who wished that a friend had said that they needed to lose weight, stop drinking, go back to work, or leave a spouse. But most were talking hypothetically. Only a handful of the women I spoke with said that they found such interventions helpful when they actually happened. One of these was the actress whose friend told her to do something about her weight. She said, "As hurt as I was, it was the push I needed. I started exercising, and I stopped eating all of the comfort foods that I had added to my diet while I was nursing. I don't know why I needed someone else to say it to me like that. I already knew what I needed to do. I stayed away from her for a long, long time after that comment. But in the end, I was grateful to her for giving me a kick in the butt. Even though I pulled away from her for a while, I had to admit that what she did was an act of real friendship. And eventually, I let her know how much I appreciated it."

The degree of connectedness between two women may make a difference in whether or not they can tolerate such direct, and painful, observations. We may listen to something that a good friend says that would seem unacceptable from someone less close to us. But sometimes we prefer our bad-tasting medicine from strangers.

This is how it worked for Eileen. "One of the other mothers at my son's school told me that she had decided not to send her son to camp. She said she thought it was just too long for an eight-year-old to be away from home. And that they would have the rest of their lives to be away," Eileen said. "It's funny. When she said it, I realized she was right. Somehow I could take the advice from her, but not from Lizzie — partly because I didn't trust her judgment in this case, since she had never gone to camp, but partly because it was just one of a million things she kept telling me to do or not do."

Controlling or Suggesting?

Whether you are the person feeling controlled or the one trying to do the controlling, you may find that how a suggestion is presented makes a big difference in whether or not it is accepted. Many women told me that they had learned to offer advice in a less direct, more sympathetic manner, with fairly good success. Sometimes it is the tone of voice or the amount of energy that makes a difference. During her 2016 presidential campaign, Hillary Clinton said, "Women are seen through a different lens." She said she had learned that, as a woman, she could not be as passionate, loud, or direct as a man, even if she was trying to communicate the same thing. "I'll go to these events and there will be men speaking before me, and they'll be pounding the message, and screaming about how we need to win the election. And people will love it. And I want to do the same thing. Because I care about this stuff. But I've learned that I can't be quite so passionate in my presentation. I love to wave my arms, but apparently that's a little bit scary to people. And I can't yell too much. It comes across as 'too loud' or 'too shrill' or 'too this' or 'too that.'"[9]

Patsy, a lawyer who sent me the article about Clinton, said, "This is bullshit. I tell my friends what I think, and they either like it or lump it. The ones who like it are the ones who stick around. The truth is, they always know where they stand with me. No questions." (Of course, Patsy was not running for president.)

But Trish, a petite blond pediatric dentist, said in a soft Southern accent, "I grew up with four younger siblings. I was always telling them what to do, and they'll tell you that I still do. That's just because I know what's best for all of them." She continued, "But as I got older, I realized that people respond better when you don't try to push them around. We have a saying in the South that you can catch more flies with honey than with vinegar. It means that you can get things done the way you want them done if you make it a pleasant experience. Yelling at someone, or criticizing them, or telling them all the things they've done wrong isn't going to get them to do what you know they should do." She grinned mischievously. "But telling them what a good job they're doing and then making a teeny, tiny suggestion about what they might do next . . . well, it works with my children, my sisters, my friends — and sometimes with my wife."

When friends either take or give up control, it can diminish the possibility of psychological and emotional growth on both sides of a friendship. On the other hand, as we mature and develop a stronger sense of our own identity, it can be easier to stand up to demanding friends.

For example, after her experience with Mila, Juliana stayed away from other girls. "Only after I married and had a daughter did I realize that I was missing out on something important. But for a lot of reasons I had developed a deep distrust of other women. I don't think it was all Mila's fault. I probably was also reacting to being so far from my family. And I felt so different from everyone else at school. I was very lonely, so I turned to my studies for comfort." With the birth of her child, Juliana began to make tentative connections with other women in her community. "I found one really wonderful friend," she said. "A social worker who lived in my neighborhood. Maybe because of her work, or maybe because of her personality — or maybe a little of both — she never tried to tell me what to do. She just told me stories about her own experiences, or experiences of people she knew. She introduced me to a wonderful group of women, who gradually became my friends. They're the most nurturing, supportive women in the world. But I'm still allergic to being told what to do. Everybody knows — it's kind of an in-joke — that they have to be very careful when offering advice to Juliana."

Development is not always in a positive direction. While some of us get better at standing up for ourselves, and some of us get less controlling over time, some women who were bossy when they were young get even worse as they get older. Lily, at eighty-seven, said that her friend Marguerite "has always told me what to do, from what time to put my kids to bed to what to make for my husband's dinner. Now she tells me what I should wear and what I should eat and when I should come to the community hall to play bridge." They live in the same residential community, and Lily told me that she found Marguerite's controlling behavior worse than ever. "But it doesn't bother me the way it used to," she said. "I have other friends who are much easier to be with. And I feel pretty comfortable with who I am and what I want to do these days."

She also said that she understood Marguerite better now. "I used to wonder if she was right when she said that my outfit wasn't good for a particular event." But one day another friend complimented her on an outfit that Marguerite had just criticized. "I don't like to gossip," Lily said, "but that day I couldn't help it. The words just slipped out of my mouth. I told her that I was feeling a little sensitive because of what Marguerite had said, and my friend was horrified. 'She's just jealous,' she told me. 'You look wonderful, as always. Don't listen to her!'"

Lily felt better after that, but then she got angry. "Who is she to tell me what to do?" she asked herself. "I told Marguerite I wanted to know why she thought I should do everything her way, and she said, 'Because I'm older than you and I know better.'" Lily laughed. "She's ninety-two. I'm eighty-nine. I'm wondering how much more she thinks I need to learn."

Ultimately, however, Lily forgave her friend. "She's lonely, and she's afraid she's losing her powers. Well, she is. We all are. It's part of getting older. So I let her boss me around because I think it makes her feel better, and then I ignore what she tells me to do." Lily smiled and added, "It's okay, because at our age, by the next day neither one of us remembers what she told me to do anyway."

As we have seen, similarities are important in women's friendships. They provide us with a context and a sense of connectedness. But differences add spice to friendship.

"What's really incredible about the group of women I'm involved with now," Juliana said, "is that we are all very different. And everyone supports these differences. We like being together because we learn from and grow from one another. It would be awful being part of a group where everyone's the same."

We often grow and develop as a result of input from friends who have a different take on the world or are involved in activities we have not participated in before. Finding a balance between similarity and difference is one key to both giving and accepting advice. And being able to give and accept advice without feeling controlling or controlled may be a key to healthy, meaningful friendships over time.

Liz put it this way: "I have learned, although with difficulty, that Eileen and I are not exactly the same. When I think that I know what she should be doing, I try to remind myself that I only know what *I* would do in her place. And I try, although I don't think I always succeed, to say it that way to her."

And Eileen replied, "And I have learned that I don't have to do what Lizzie wants. I don't even have to respond to her suggestion at all, though that always gets her a little steamed. The best response tends to be to thank her and to tell her I'll think about it, and then, after a beat, to say something like, 'I know it's what you would do. I'm just not sure it's what I need to do.' She gets that now and, although she will usually push her point a little more, I can stand my ground. And she will eventually let go."

What You Can Do

There are times when we seek advice from friends, but instead of receiving good counsel, we end up with unwanted proposals that interfere with our own ability to problem-solve. At other times, when we just want to complain, a friend takes that as an opportunity to tell us what to do. In either case, it is important to communicate what you really need from your friend. And while you are clarifying what you want from her, you may also need to set some boundaries.

Many of us have difficulty setting boundaries, so when a friend gets a little (or a lot) overbearing in her advice giving, we are not always comfortable with pushing back even a little. And this discomfort can lead us to give in when we don't want to. It can also provoke an overreaction, such as the time when, after Liz made a minor suggestion, Eileen burst out with "Why don't you just mind your own business for once!" "I was so embarrassed," Eileen said. "That's not like me at all. But I guess I got the point across. Lizzie was stunned into total silence for the first time since I've known her!"

There is a lot of advice available for those of us who have difficulty saying no.[10] Much of it boils down to not taking the other person's behavior personally. If you can see the advice in perspective, you don't have to take it to heart, and you might even find some of it useful. It's helpful to consider where the advice is coming from — for example, your friend may have good intentions, but she does not really understand the situation. Or you may observe that your friend's intentions are not completely good, as when Lily realized that Marguerite's advice and criticism often came from a sense of insecurity and loneliness. "I'm a big girl," Lily said. "I don't have to do what she says. And I don't have to take her advice to heart. She's got her own problems. And they aren't related to whether or not my dress looks nice, or I've got on too much makeup, or I'm allowed to wear white pants after Labor Day or any of the other crazy fashion rules she believes we're supposed to follow."

Here are two important things to remember before giving advice: (1) listen carefully, and (2) ask yourself if the advice you want to give is anything your friend has not heard before.

Listening is not as easy as many of us think. Mental health professionals have described two very different forms of usefully hearing what your friend is saying. One is "reflective listening," which means that you reflect back what you are hearing your friend say, without adding anything to it. But sometimes just saying back what your friend is saying is not enough. You need to let her know that you are thinking about and understanding what she is telling you. This kind of listening is called "active listening," and involves your responding in ways that communicate your understanding of some of the complexities of her situation.

On a terrific *Psychology Today* blog about giving advice, Meg Selig,[11] author of the book *Changepower!: 37 Secrets to Habit Change Success,* suggests three important tools for active listening: (1) expressing empathy for the other person's situation, (2) telling stories that show your understanding (for instance, a story about a similar situation in your own life), and (3) acknowledging that your friend should take any advice you give with a grain of salt, since even though you are sympathetic, you cannot completely know what she is feeling or what all of the details of the situation might be.

Sometimes it's better not to give advice at all, though. The psychologist Thomas Plante tells us, "Advice giving usually doesn't work, and often completely backfires."[12] But if you genuinely feel that what you have to say is important, useful, and something your friend hasn't heard before, it is crucial to communicate that you do not think you have all of the answers. Be tentative, suggests Meg Selig. Advice communicated in the spirit of not knowing everything can help a friend grow, but advice given as superior knowledge can feel condescending. The only thing that will grow from that sort of advice is resentment, insecurity, and very possibly rebellion. Your friend might do the opposite of what you suggest, just to show you that you are not in control.

Whether you are ninety-two, twenty-two, or somewhere in between, remember that both receiving and giving advice are complicated. A person's motivation to offer advice may be genuinely openhearted or selfish or somewhere in between — and the person may not understand her own motivation. Likewise, it may be hard for you to figure out what lies behind your desire to suggest to a friend what she should do. And even the closest friend can sometimes give you bad counsel or feel controlled or criticized when you offer well-meaning suggestions.

Still, even with these potential pitfalls, it is possible to find a sense of balance concerning friendship and advice. At eighty-seven, Lily seemed to have found it. She said, "Marguerite might want to take control of my life because she can't control her own; but she's also got a good heart. She thinks she's right and she wants me to have the benefit of her so-called knowledge. I try to remember that it comes from a good place. But that doesn't mean I have to do what she says."

8

~

With Friends like This,
Who Needs Enemies?

COMPETITION BETWEEN FRIENDS

S EO-YUN WAS A SUCCESSFUL ADVERTISING ACCOUNT
manager who was popular with her staff and had a large
group of friends. Her husband was also doing well in his business, and the two of them enjoyed a life that was the envy of many
of their friends. They had three adorable children, a house in the
suburbs, and a second home in the mountains. And she had a secret
that was destroying her happiness.

Unlike most of her women friends, Seo-yun did not watch her
diet. Other women would look on enviously as she sparkled her way
through any gathering, eating and drinking heartily and encourag-
ing everyone else to do the same. But she had never told anyone, not

her closest friend or even her husband, that she was suffering from an eating disorder. She could not stop eating once she started. After a dinner party or business lunch she would buy more food and continue to eat until she was so stuffed that she could barely breathe. She would force herself to throw up and then fall into a deep, almost drugged sleep. The next morning she would wake up hating herself.

Seo-yun's problem, like most eating disorders, probably resulted from a combination of biological, psychological, emotional, cultural, and historical factors.[1] For Seo-yun, as for many women, a wish to please others, a drive for perfection, and cultural, family, and peer pressure to be thin all contributed to her out-of-control behavior. "I come from a very competitive world," she said. "From very early I learned that I had to be the prettiest, the thinnest, the smartest, and the most successful in order to be okay. I work hard to be all of those things. But what no one told me was that if you are the best, then everyone will hate you. No one will be your friend!"

Although most of her friends said how happy they were for her, Seo-yun knew that some of them resented her picture-perfect life. "They say I'm lucky, which of course is true. But they don't see how hard I work. I had a good girlfriend who broke up with me because she said everything came so easily to me. I had to laugh. *Nothing* comes easily, but I think I am supposed to make it look that way." She added, "But making it look easy creates problems that no one tells you about. Korean women are very physical. We hold hands and take each other's arms in public. We look like we're so close. This friend did that with me. But then she told me that we couldn't be friends anymore. Just like that."

Like many women, Seo-yun had never imagined that her friends might envy her. "What would they envy me for?" she wondered. "I don't want them to feel bad. I admire my friends, and I see all the things they have that I don't have. In myself, I just see my faults." She was simply on a mission to improve herself, or at least that is how she saw it. I heard much the same thing from many of the women I talked with, so I started asking how they understood this phenomenon. Why are women so blind to competition and envy from other women? A senior executive in her fifties said, "I think women all over the world are still trained to doubt themselves. Put that together with our need to please, and you get even the smartest, most capable women feeling insecure. How could we ever imagine that someone would think we had more than they do?"

The area in which women were most open about competing concerned men. After divorcing her husband, Daphne heard from other women that Jennifer had always envied her. "I don't think of myself as someone anybody would envy," Daphne told me. "I'm a big, awkward, funny-looking woman, and I was a big, awkward, funny-looking girl. I'm not particularly smart or accomplished. What's there to envy?"

For many women, the feeling that we have nothing for anyone else to envy is closely linked to a difficulty with accepting compliments. There is an old joke that a woman may take hours getting dressed, but if you compliment what she is wearing, she will respond not with "Thank you," but with a self-deprecating comment like "What, this old rag? I just pulled anything I could put my hands on out of my closet." This denial of value, whether concerning our job, our house, or our appearance, combined with disbelief that anyone really admires us, can color our friendships in surprising ways. Like the old Groucho Marx joke, "I wouldn't belong to a club that would have me as a member," women sometimes fall into the trap of believing that anyone who chooses to be our friend must be flawed — otherwise that person would not want to be friends with us.

I have heard many variations of this downplaying of our own achievements and positive qualities, so many variations that I began digging more deeply into their roots. The psychologist Adrienne Harris tells us that what I was seeing is not unusual. She says that despite changes in attitude toward women and competition in some cultures in recent decades, many of us continue to feel uncomfortable when competitive issues surface in our relationships with other women.[2] Ruth Moulton, who wrote about women's psychological issues in the 1970s, explained that the qualities of pride, aggression, and self-regard that go along with success were, at the time, antithetical to feelings of femininity, which were associated with selflessness, nurturing, and modesty.[3] Harris, like many of the women I spoke with, says that these conflicts are alive and well today. They often play an important, albeit silent, role in women's friendships.

Competition? What Competition?

One of the ways that competition affects friendships is through denial of its existence. Even among the youngest women I have talked with, it seems that competitive, envious, and jealous feelings are hard for many women to manage in general, and particularly difficult in friendships, where we expect — and are expected — to be supportive and caring above everything else. So we simply refuse to admit these feelings exist. Many of the women I spoke with were surprised when I asked them about feelings of envy and competitiveness in their friendships. "My friends and I adore each other," said one lithe yoga teacher, echoing the sentiments of numerous others. "We take care of each other and are happy with each other's successes. We would never compete with one another."

This attitude permeates the world in which we live. One woman who had managed to have a successful career under a regime that is highly intolerant of women who worked in any position outside their homes told me that an older woman friend of her mother's had been a role model and a support throughout her career. "She was just incredible to me," she said, with tears in her eyes. "She was advisor, mentor, and confidante. When I got downhearted, she boosted me. When I succeeded, she celebrated with me." When I asked if she had ever felt that there were any competitive or envious aspects of their relationship, she looked at me in surprise. "No," she said, "I never felt anything like that." She may, of course, have been right. Competitive feelings do not exist everywhere, and mentors often get so much satisfaction and self-esteem from the relationship with their mentees that they do not feel competitive with them. But Deborah Tannen tells us that even in supportive connections, conversations can sometimes contain "a subtle or not so subtle competitive edge."[4]

Sally, a musician in her sixties who supplemented the income she made from performances by teaching, told me that she once had a student who was clearly on her way to stardom. "I loved working with her," Sally said. "But I couldn't help myself. Every so often I felt angry at her because she was going to have all of the success that I had wanted." We do not always recognize these competitive feelings for what they are, since we frequently push them away before we even become fully conscious of them. The unfortunate result is that they sometimes emerge indirectly, in anger or a hypercritical attitude, which in turn can lead to other difficulties.

In her book *Lean In,* Sheryl Sandberg acknowledges the history of women's hostile competitiveness with one another in business — one fictional example is the aggressive, merciless female executive played by Meryl Streep in *The Devil Wears Prada.* But Sandberg tells us that this attitude existed mostly in the past. Nowadays, she writes, women are eagerly supporting their female colleagues, not undermining them in order to protect their own success.[5] Yet many women have described a different experience. As Susie Orbach and Luise Eichenbaum put it, the "sisterhood" image of women's friendships sometimes obscures the complex and occasionally hurtful feelings that are also part of these relationships.[6]

A successful businesswoman who is active in an organization

that supports young female entrepreneurs and potential executives told me that she found men more trustworthy than women. "They're just more open about competing. And they don't take it so personally. Women get all sneaky and manipulative and mean. It's like they don't want to admit that they're competing, so they go underground. And then it gets downright ugly. Men will be friends with you even if you are competing the hell with each other. They're just straightforward about it. That's why I prefer to be friends with men."

In many cultures women have entered the highly competitive worlds of sports, business, and a variety of professions. And yet many of these women I spoke with agreed that men are better able to incorporate competition into their friendships. They pointed to stories of men who compete at work and then go out and have a great time together at the end of the day. "Women just don't do that," said one thirty-something businesswoman. A former college athlete said, "When we were playing as teammates we were all very supportive of each other. But when you separated us, there was lots of snarkiness. We could be real bitches."

The *Vogue* writer Rebecca Johnson reports that male athletes are often good buddies with their biggest competitors, while women seem to have a harder time with this. She says, "Roger Federer might have dinner with Stan Wawrinka after a match, but among the women, it's mostly the cold shoulder." She goes on to describe Serena Williams's close friendships with her fiercest competitors. Williams told her, "It's hard and lonely at the top. That's why it's so fun to have Caroline [Wozniacki], and my sister [Venus], too."[7]

All's Fair in Love

When it comes to love, women are sometimes a little more open about their competitiveness. Many women I spoke with complained about friends who deserted them when they got involved with a man, but most also said that they understood. "Finding the man you're going to marry is probably one of the most important jobs we have," said one recently married twenty-nine-year-old. Competing for another woman's man is not exactly accepted, but many women understand it far better than stealing someone else's job. Daphne said, "I can't accept what Jennifer did, and I blame Mike as well. But I do understand. Mike was pretty special — or at least that's what I thought. I always thought I was so lucky to have him, and I totally understood why she wanted him too. I just thought she cared too much about me to do something so destructive."

But many women have a hard time being direct about competitive situations of any nature. Rose, a teacher in her late twenties, told me that her best friend had just gotten engaged. "I'm thrilled for her," she said. "I love her fiancé and I love seeing them so happy together. But sometimes when I'm with them, I feel bad. I love the idea that she found someone, and it makes me feel like there's hope for me. But I feel like she kind of looks down on me. It's very subtle, but it's like she's thinking, 'I found someone. What's wrong with you that you haven't found anyone?' It makes me want to stay away. I don't talk to her about how I feel so much anymore."

An attractive brunette in her forties said, "When I got divorced some of my women friends stopped having me over to dinner with their husbands. I know they were afraid I was going to make a play for one of them. I wouldn't have. But for sure I would have flirted with them. I just needed to know they found me attractive. I don't think it's such a terrible thing, but I get it that it made my friends nervous. So they excluded me." And twenty-five-year-old Tracey said, "My friend Joanna is always dragging me out to bars. I wouldn't mind it, except that anytime a cute woman starts to talk to me, Joanna moves in on her immediately. Joanna and I are just buddies, but it seems like she can't stand it if another woman is interested in me."

In her fictional account of a tightly knit community of women in biblical times, Anita Diamant describes a world of women in which a heroine is fully aware of her own envious and competitive feelings toward her best friend and other women as well.[8] Often the competition in these relationships was over husbands, some of whom were shared by several women. In Diamant's fictional world, there is a clear hierarchy partly determined by marital status (with unmarried women at the bottom), partly by the position a husband holds in the male community, and partly by who is best loved by a shared husband. Competition for power, respect, and love is openly acknowledged.

In the real world today, some religions view angry and hostile actions between female community members as sin. Yet several women I spoke to who had grown up in closed religious communities said that they felt the women there dealt with competitive feelings more openly than women did in the secular world. "If a friend got something you wanted," said one woman, "whether it was a man, a dress or piece of cloth, a book, or a piece of fruit, you could have it out with her. You could call her names, or you could sulk. You could even stop having anything to do with her for a while. Some of the older women would eventually call you out on it, and you would have to figure out a way to make up. But your feelings were your feelings."

"One-Downsmanship"

Many women allow themselves to compete openly only in a way that is almost a contradiction in terms. This is "one-downsmanship," a competition in which the winner is the person who can present herself as the biggest loser: "Why would anyone feel competitive with me? I'm the worst, the unhappiest, the most unsuccessful, or the ugliest of anyone I know."

There are two big problems with one-downsmanship. First, when it is genuine, it indicates a self-loathing that makes it difficult for others to engage with you. And second, it can sound (and sometimes is) false. This level of self-deprecation can seem like an attempt to get others to tell you how wonderful you really are. But one-downsmanship may also be a way of saying, "I'm really worse off than you are and so no threat to you." I asked women about these instances of "humble-bragging," and many immediately recognized them as something they and their friends often did. There were many variations on the "this old rag" response, including, "Really, you like my new haircut? I hate it!" An office manager said, "Women I report to, who make a lot more money and have a lot more power than I do, tell me things like 'I'm so stupid' and 'You're a genius at this kind of thing' when what they mean is 'Don't be mad at me' or 'I need your help, so be nice to me.'"

Sometimes the behavior is so subtle we don't notice it. Perhaps not surprisingly, many of the older women I spoke with were far more aware of the role of one-downsmanship in their lives. For instance, a woman in her late fifties said, "You know, I didn't realize what that was about till I got older. Women have a hard time letting friends know that we are proud of something we've done. We're afraid we'll hurt their feelings or make them jealous. But one of the great things about getting older is that I don't worry about that so much anymore. If a woman is going to be my friend, she's going to have to like herself enough to be able to be pleased with me when I'm successful."

Hiding Your Strengths

Why would you need to hide your strengths from your friends? It almost seems to be a contradiction in terms, since friends are supposed to be strong for one another. Yet many women do precisely this. We downplay our strengths in front of our friends, to protect them and to protect ourselves.

Many of the women I spoke with said that they sometimes hid their successes from friends in order not to make friends feel bad about themselves. Others told me that they were aware that if their friends resented them too much, it would destroy their relationship. But often competition and envy take a far more confusing and indirect path. Seo-yun, for example, whose friends openly envied her, learned in therapy that her eating disorder allowed her to have success and failure at the same time. "Nobody knew how unhappy I really was," she said. "But I knew. And somehow, that made it okay that I was doing so well. Secretly, I could tell myself that I was suffering as much as any of them. So I didn't have to feel bad about having things they didn't have."

We know that a good friend can make us feel normal in the midst of chaos, confusion, and self-doubt. "I know how you feel" or "I know — I do the same thing" may be some of the most calming words a woman can hear. Yet it seems that competitive strivings can interfere with our ability to give and receive such support.

Competitive feelings — that we feel toward a friend and that a friend feels toward us — can interfere with our good feelings about ourselves. Rose, the teacher with the newly engaged friend, had competitive and envious feelings that made her feel doubly bad about herself. She said, "I don't like feeling like there's something wrong with me, and I know she's not doing that on purpose. It's my own self-doubt, I'm sure. But I also don't like feeling envious of what she has. It's not the me I like to be. So I'm tempted to stay away from her because I don't want to feel like that. And that makes me feel bad too. I don't want to stay away from my good friend, and especially if it's because I'm jealous of what she has!"

Competition and envy can silently invade and destroy a relationship. Jo, whose good friend secretly went after a job that

Jo had been working toward for months, was upset about losing the job itself, but even worse, she said, was the feeling that her friend had gone after it without telling her. "I found out from my boss. That's crazy. Now I just feel like I can't trust that friend anymore."

Competition and Admiration

A soft-spoken doctoral student said, "I have known for most of my professional life that other women were competitive with me. That makes sense. We are competing for a limited number of jobs in our field. But what I don't understand is why women seem to mix up competing for something with not liking each other."

Many other women shared this concern. For Jo, it raised questions about her friend — "it made me wonder if she had ever liked me at all." And Eileen, who has been friends with Liz since high school, told me, "When we were in our twenties, Lizzie, who can be a little too direct for her own good, once got into trouble with one of her women bosses. Lizzie is super-smart and capable, and she doesn't suffer fools gladly. This woman was just not as efficient as Lizzie, and instead of acknowledging it and joining forces with her, she did everything she could to make Liz's life miserable. I'm sure Lizzie wasn't going out of her way to be extra accommodating to this woman, like everyone else did. That's just not in her nature. But it was the only time in her life that a boss seemed to really dislike her. Her brother (my boyfriend at the time) and I both tried to make her see that the woman was envious and competitive, but Lizzie kept saying, 'I haven't done anything wrong. There's no reason for her to compete with me.' She couldn't get it out of her head that if her boss was competitive with her, it meant she'd done something wrong."

Conflicting feelings about competition affect men as well as women. The British psychoanalyst Adam Phillips says that neither success nor failure is ever a "pure experience," since men and women sometimes worry that winning a competition brings the danger of losing a positive connection with someone they like or care about.[9]

Rachel Terrill, the wife of a former professional American football player, says that players' wives provided important support for one another. But she sometimes wondered if it was healthy for them to spend time together. Because their husbands often competed for the same positions, she writes, "One player's success often meant another player would lose his job. How close can our friendships be if we don't always wish the other players well? . . . Could we in friendship hurt the team?"[10]

Yet I heard repeatedly from women all over the world that most of the time when they felt competitive toward someone, it was because she had something they admired. Is there room for competitive admiration in friendship?

Janine, a forty-eight-year-old partner in a law firm, told me that she and her closest friend, Linda, a medical researcher, were longtime competitors. "We were roommates in college," she said. "We competed about everything—grades, looks, boys, sports, and anything else that was important to us. Sometimes she won, and sometimes I did. We would get angry about losing, of course. But whether we won or lost, we always cared about each other."

I asked Janine what kept the competition from hurting their friendship. "We have always been there for each other," she said. "We celebrate wins and mourn losses together." Linda supported Janine through breast cancer, and Janine was with Linda when she lost a child. "We trust each other and we know that we'll never intentionally hurt each other. We can talk about anything. We also respect and admire each other.

"We probably both did better in school than we would have if we hadn't known each other, because we were competing to get better grades and a better GPA. My being a senior partner at my firm is partly the result of my wanting to win in our never-ending competition. We're in different fields, so it's not a one-to-one correlation, but I bet if you asked her, she'd say the same thing about her own professional successes, of which there have been many. But there are things Linda can do that I'd love to be able to do and never will. She's much more generous than I am, for example. She'd give you her only coat if you were cold. I'd never do that, but those things that we admire push us to do better ourselves. I'm more generous now than when I first met Linda because I want to be more like her. I'd say our competition with each other has made us better friends —and better people too."

Competing Moms

Interestingly, one of the areas in which women often allow themselves to compete has to do with children and family. Proudly bragging about a child's accomplishments, while not always good form, feels more acceptable to many women than talking about their own accomplishments. We are used to parents showing off their children, for instance, when they get into a good college, win an award, get a part in a play, snag a prestigious job, or become a doctor or lawyer. Some women proudly describe their children's financial success, while others do this indirectly by talking about the huge new house purchased by a son or daughter, and all of its exquisite decorations. Even here, though, humble-bragging can arise. One woman told me of a former friend who always put her son and daughter-in-law down. "But you could tell that she wanted you to say how wonderful whatever they had done really was. She was completely fake about the whole thing. It was just her upside-down way of bragging about her kids."

Even tiny accomplishments can become part of the competitive interplay between mom friends. One young woman, aware of the competitive nature of these friendships and of her wish not to hurt anyone in her circle of friends, told me, "When my baby sat up by herself before my friends' babies did, I was so proud. I didn't say anything, of course, since I didn't want to make them feel bad."

She understood that the indirect communication would be, "I am such a good mother/person/woman because I have such a good/successful/athletic/smart/child." And that this would stir up simultaneous feelings of inferiority and resentment in other women. "When I hear my friends talk about their kids' social lives, I worry that my daughter isn't one of the popular kids," said a mother of a seven-year-old. When I asked why she saw that as a problem, she said, "I wasn't popular. I always felt hurt and left out. It was very bad for my self-esteem. I want my daughter to feel good about herself." She was reliving her own social anxieties through her daughter, and living them out at the same time with her own friends.

Subtle and not-so-subtle put-downs are part of the competitive underworld of many of these relationships. In some communities, for example, stay-at-home mothers worry that their working friends see them as inferior; yet many working mothers told me that they got clear messages from their friends that it was not good for their children to spend so much time with a babysitter or in daycare. These often unacknowledged but oh-so-common "friend competitions" play a central role in Liane Moriarty's *Big Little Lies*, where the putdowns are subtle and complex. One mother in the book, supposedly complimenting another for staying home with her children, says, "I'm the sort of person who would be bored out of my mind if I had to be a full-time mother." But the other woman clearly understands the not-so-subtle communication that "Renata was the smart one, the one who needed more mental stimulation, because she had a career."[11]

Jealousy and Envy

Psychoanalytic theory generally defines envy as the feeling that someone else has something that you find desirable; this feeling is often accompanied by a wish to take that desirable something away from the other person or to destroy their ability to enjoy it. Jealousy occurs when one in a group of three feels excluded or rejected by one or both of the other two.[12] In popular terms, however, many of the women I have spoken with viewed envy as somehow less hurtful or destructive than jealousy. As one thirty-two-year-old organic farmer told me, "Jealousy makes you suspicious and doubtful of someone you love, whether it's your lover or your spouse, and that's a terrible feeling."

Jealousy is not so distant from sibling rivalry, the competition between siblings for a parent's love, affection, or admiring words. Samantha, a shy, quiet woman, told me that her large group of friends was the most important thing in her life. "My friend Mimi brought me into the group," she said. "She's the mover and shaker in the group, in fact. Without her, we wouldn't exist. She's the one who starts a lot of the activities we do together. She'll say to someone, 'Let's get the gang together for pizza night,' and that person starts the text chain. Everybody loves Mimi, and everybody wants to be her best friend. There's this unacknowledged competition to show how well we know her, or how special we are to her. And there are sometimes unpleasant catfights between some of us when we feel left out of her inner circle."

In her book *When Friendship Hurts,* the sociologist Jan Yager[13] tells us that a threesome of friends can be nurturing and support-ive, but it can also be problematic. While such a grouping can some-times be easier than a twosome, it has the potential for jealousy and conflict. Preethi, the thirty-six-year-old radiologist who worked hard to see the positive in all of her friends, told me that she had once been close with two women. "We did everything together," she said. "But then one of them started to complain that I spent more time with the other. She was jealous of our relationship and started doing mean things to drive us apart. Like, she would gossip about one of us to the other. Or she would complain about something one of us had done. We finally had to stop being friends with her alto-gether. It was kind of sad, and I felt bad, but there didn't seem to be any other solution."

When these dark feelings damage a close relationship, you may feel like your only choice is to end the friendship. But the psycho-analyst Virginia Demos, who has spent much of her career studying emotions, tells us that we have to make room for feelings that we identify as "bad" as well as for those we see as "good."[14] Finding a way to integrate competition and rivalry with loving, admiring, and nurturing feelings toward the same person can be difficult, but ex-tremely rewarding.

What You Can Do

There is an old saying that imitation is the highest form of flattery. What many — not all, of course — men seem to understand that we women sometimes don't is that competition is also flattery. Who competes with someone over something we don't like, care about, or want for ourselves? And in the end, what many women have not yet figured out is that honest competition can be good for our self-esteem and for our friendships. If a friend is good enough to compete with, then she is also someone we can admire, appreciate, and learn from. Still, many women have a way to go before they can be friends with their competitors.

The good news is that you can learn to integrate competitive feelings into close relationships. It may take time and work, but it's worth giving your friends and yourself a chance. First, of course, you will need to acknowledge the feelings and stop seeing them as something bad. Pat Summitt, the former coach of the University of Tennessee's women's basketball team, who won more games than any other NCAA Division I basketball coach, male or female, probably understood what went into healthy competition better than most women. She once said, "There is always someone better than you. Whatever it is that you do for a living, chances are, you will run into a situation in which you are not as talented as the person next to you. That's when being a competitor can make a difference in your fortunes."[15]

Kim, a thirty-two-year-old marketing director, told me that she and her best friend were also competitive. "We love each other," she said. "And I don't think we compete exactly the same way that guys do. Sometimes we don't realize what's happening until we get into an argument, and then one of us will laugh and say, 'Oh, I just wanted to be better than you on this one.' And the other one will always say, 'You're so good at so many things, could you let me win this time?' And that will be the end of the argument and whatever bad feelings were going on."

A number of women said that they felt less competitive as they got older. But many told me that they had learned to find other women who were comfortable with who they were; they didn't try to outdo one another or hide their successes. A writer in her late sixties told me, "I finally got close to women when I was living my adult life. We were raising kids together, and I just began to feel trust. I found a group of strong women who felt good about themselves. They weren't competitive, they were just wonderful people who were interested, curious, and had a strong sense of identity. They weren't struggling to be smarter, to get ahead, prettier. Judgment was lessened."

The feminist psychoanalysts Susie Orbach and Luise Eichenbaum offer this image of the kinds of relationships women can aspire to: "honest, loving relationships built not on fear, betrayal, competition or envy, and not in solidarity in opposition to men, but on sharing, contact between equals, and support for autonomy."[16] A number of women told me that they had found friends who were comfortable with competing. "We just don't see it as all or nothing," said one woman who was a rower in college and is in a highly competitive tennis league as an adult. "Whether you win or you lose, whether you play a lousy game or an excellent one, none of it changes who you are as a person. There are some women who get so tied up in their game that they forget that lesson. But," she laughed, "the group I play with won't let anybody get away with that. Everybody has strengths and everybody has weaknesses. If we can't work that into our relationships, then we can't enjoy winning."

Mary McCarthy's novel *The Group* tells the story of eight young women, from their graduation from Vassar College through their early adult years and, eventually, the death of one of their group. As we follow their tangled paths through romance and heartbreak, career, marriage, and babies, we also get to see the complicated role of rivalry in their friendships. Libby, for instance, is painfully aware of conflicting feelings of envy and pity for her friend Polly, when she finds her living in genteel poverty. Thinking about the handmade Christmas gift she had received from her friend, Libby goes from criticism to admiration. "Actually, those pomander balls were quite snazzy; they were a very original Christmas present and cost practically nothing."[17]

The more directly we acknowledge these feelings, the less likely it is that we will resort to underhanded or manipulative behavior when they emerge — sparing us toxic feelings and damage to our self-esteem *and* our friendships.

But questions of jealousy and rivalry inevitably get us thinking about romantic relationships. As we discuss the question of sexuality in women's friendships, we will consider another aspect of competition, envy, jealousy, and rivalry.

9

⁓

Sexual Tension in Women's Friendships

CCORDING TO SOME FEMINIST THEORISTS, LOVE and friendship may not be as distinct as we imagine.[1] Yet when sexual tension emerges in a relationship between women friends, the usual fear of rejection is complicated by cultural taboos against homosexuality and lesbianism.

Courageous television personalities such as Ellen DeGeneres and Rosie O'Donnell helped pave the way, at least in some places, for more open discussion of romantic love between two women. Suddenly, just like famous heterosexual couples, popular lesbian couples and details of their romances filled gossip magazines and became commonplace household conversation. Recently, an ad for

Sainsbury's supermarkets in Great Britain celebrated same-sex parenting, and in the United States, a Zales jewelry ad showed two women becoming engaged. Television programs, from *Rosewood* to *Degrassi* to *Orphan Black,* explore in ever-greater depth the complexities, pain, humor, and joy of romantic love between two women.

The main characters of the television series *Sex and the City* once briefly considered and then discarded the possibility of mutual romantic attraction, but an undercurrent of sexual tension between the women plays quietly in the background in many episodes. Like many contemporary women, Carrie and her friends are highly conflicted about their looks, their attractiveness, and their sexuality, sometimes flaunting their bodies and sometimes hiding them.[2] As is true in many women's friendships, sexuality, jealousy, and competition are often commingled yet not openly discussed.

Even today, when fluidity of sexual identity is acknowledged and freedom to choose a sexual partner of any gender is allowed, at least in some places, the issue of sex and friendship between women can still disturb. Consider the famous kisses between Madonna, Britney Spears, and Christina Aguilera at the MTV Video Music Awards in 2003, which caused outrage. Madonna, who says that she is bisexual, told one interviewer that she has had a lot of crushes on women but has only been in love with men. Christina, on the other hand, says that she is straight but finds women "hornier to look at" than men.[3]

She is not alone. In one recent study, almost three-quarters of the straight women participants were stimulated sexually by looking at other women.[4] What impact do these sexual responses have on friendships?

In some cases, they are simply part of our connection as friends. Research confirms that women are often sexually aroused by touching and being touched.[5] Yet such contact does not necessarily translate into sexual interest or a sense of feeling comfortable with your body. For example, Seo-yun, a slender, delicately built woman, said that although in her native South Korea women are physically affectionate in public and in private, it's not sexual. When I asked if Seo-yun thought the physical contact with other women had helped her feel better about herself physically, she laughed. "Absolutely not. I have suffered all my life from feeling inadequate and imperfect. No matter what I accomplish, I feel like a failure. I am working on this problem. And my body is part of the problem."

Melody, on the other hand, is one of many women who told me that they became more comfortable with their body and their heterosexuality through a brief foray into a sexual relationship with a good female friend. A thirty-five-year-old kindergarten teacher, she lived in the Midwest with her boyfriend and their two children. "I'm very lucky," she said. "I have really, really close girlfriends from every period of my life. I would go so far as to say that my friendships, more than anything else in my life, have shaped and formed me. I'm still ridiculously close to my two best friends from childhood. One is more like a sister than anything. And the other one — well, when we were younger, we experimented with each other sexually. All through adolescence, sometimes while we were also having relationships with guys, we experimented together. We love each other deeply and have talked about wishing that we could be romantic together, but we don't feel that way about each other. But I know that I am who I am today because of this relationship. We understand each other more deeply and truly than anyone else in the world."

A pale-skinned, freckled woman in her forties who had recently separated from her husband of twenty years said, "I was having a glass of wine with a group of really good friends. They're all smart, successful, and so interesting, but also very different from one another. After the usual chitchat, we started talking about sexual experiences in college. One of them, who has been happily married to a great guy for twenty-five years, said that she and her college roommate had played around with each other, kissing, touching, giving each other orgasms. Almost all of the other women around the table said they had done some of that too. I didn't know about this when I was in college! I had no idea that it was going on. Where was I? What was wrong with me? I was so naive then, I might have been horrified, which might be why no one ever suggested it to me. But I think it might have made a huge difference in my life. Not that I would have found out that I was gay. I really like sex with a man. But I might have learned to be more comfortable with my body."

Dr. Suzanna Rose, a researcher specializing in the psychology of women's relationships, says that even when two friends are heterosexual, there can be a physical link between them. She says that love and friendship are "two discrete yet inextricably intertwined concepts, each relying on the other for full expression."[6] Research has shown that in women's brains, sexual desire and lust are frequently connected to our sense of safety.[7] And we often feel safest with our friends. So, even when we have no interest in becoming sexual with a close woman friend, we might have some sexual stirrings when we are around her. One twenty-six-year-old said, "Living with women roommates, you learn all about their bodily functions. You get comfortable with those things in them and in yourself, because you just don't have a choice." A retired physician in her seventies told me that when she was in medical school, she and her friends "would sit around with mirrors and our copies of the book *Our Bodies, Ourselves,* which had just been published, and look at our vaginas together." She said that it was not particularly sexual, but rather "a safe way to get to know our bodies."

Despite the benefits of today's greater openness to different varieties of sexual experience, this freedom does have a dark side. A recent college grad told me, "I went to a school where everyone was hooking up with everyone else. You were supposed to be open to anything and everything. I didn't really like it. I'm not attracted to women and I didn't want to have sex with my women friends. But there was a culture of snobbery about anyone who didn't open herself up to it." While research has suggested that the popular concept of "lesbian until graduation" may be more fantasy than reality, there is also data suggesting that one of the causes of the binge-drinking epidemic on college campuses around the world is the pressure to conform to the "hookup culture" at school and university.[8]

The pressure to be open to a range of sexual experiences has apparently had an interesting surprise impact on young people. According to some studies, people in their late teens and early twenties are less likely to have sex now than the same age group two decades ago.[9] Does this mean they are less comfortable with their bodies? Perhaps not, but the evidence seems to suggest that greater sexual and gender fluidity, in combination with a widespread "hookup culture," may be leading to more, rather than less, discomfort with our bodies.

When One Wants Sex and the Other Does Not

Understanding, mutuality, and equality are often foundational to deeply meaningful connections between women, whether sexual or not. Yet sexual tensions can cause equality and mutuality to go out the window. Emma Straub beautifully illustrates the difficulty of dealing with a one-sided attraction in her novel *Modern Lovers,* in which three women struggle to negotiate conflicts between their mutual but imperfectly balanced lust, love, and friendship.[10] Research into women's sexuality has shown that women are aroused by empathy or identification — that is, by imagining what someone we care about is feeling in her body.[11] Such empathy is a key component of friendship between women. The feeling does not necessarily confirm sexual preference or gender identity, but finding a safe relationship in which to explore some of your responses can be a pathway to greater self-knowledge.

For instance, Francesca and Andrea told me about their very different ways of learning about their sexuality. Francesca was in her late forties and worked as a magazine editor. Andrea, who was thirty-nine, was an IT specialist. They had two children, two dogs, and a hamster. "We got married five years ago," said Francesca. "When we were growing up, that wasn't even a possibility, two women marrying, so I can't say it was the culmination of a lifetime dream. But it was — still is — pretty amazing."

"I always had a lot of friends, growing up," said Andrea, "but it was painful being a girl who was interested in other girls sexually. I knew pretty early in my life that I was attracted to other girls. Not all of my friends understood, and of course some girls weren't comfortable with it. One of the hardest things for me was figuring out which girls were 'just friends,' which ones were experimenting, and which ones were into other girls, like me. But I usually did figure it out."

"Yeah, that's definitely not how it was for me," added Francesca. "Growing up in Latin America, where there's a lot of physical touching, but sex between girls was definitely not okay, it was difficult to accept who I was and difficult to figure out who I could share my feelings with. I learned the hard way to read the nonverbal signals that other girls put out. I was a teenager, and I was madly in love with my best friend. We were so close, I thought she knew who I was and felt the same way. But when I approached her sexually, she was horrified. She told me not to speak to her ever again. I still cry over that sometimes." Andrea put her arm around Francesca's shoulders.

Another difficulty for many women is that in many cultures, love and friendship are viewed as two separate sets of feelings. So when one friend feels romantic and another wants to keep the relationship platonic, what happens to the friendship? A number of women spoke of this conundrum. One mother of two told me of a good friend who had been married and had children. "And then she realized that she was more attracted to women than to men. I was totally okay with that, but when she said she was attracted to me, I felt like that was crossing a line I didn't want to cross." A psychologist told a similar story. "I was very close friends with a colleague at work. When she came out, she wanted to get involved with me sexually. But I loved her as a friend, not a romantic interest. It was hard, but we worked it out. We decided we could stay friends and not have to turn the relationship into a sexual one. We're both married now, and she and her wife and my husband and I are all very close."

For some women, sexual expression simply flows as part of daily life. A professional dancer told me, "Ours is such a physical profession, we use our bodies all of the time. Of course we're going to be sexual. I have had affairs with men and women who I dance with. It's about friendship and connection and physicality. You just have to make sure it doesn't interfere with your work. If it gets romantic, that's when it can be a problem." But not everyone agrees about this. Another dancer told me, "In my business we touch each other all the time, but it's not sexual. It's our work. To get sexual would be distracting. It's not where we go."

Friendships with Guys

It is a widely held belief that men and women cannot be friends. "Somebody will end up getting hurt," your mom may have told you when you were young and wanted to hang out with your best guy friend. Guy-and-girl best friends who fall painfully in — and out of — love, often in secret, sometimes humorously and sometimes with devastating results, have been a recurring theme in popular books, movies, plays, and television shows. Romantic comedies of best friends who fall in love, from old favorites like *When Harry Met Sally* to the more recent *Friends with Benefits,* stoke our fantasies of platonic friendships that morph into true love.

"My best friends were always boys," says an Israeli accountant in her thirties. "It's not that I didn't like girls, but I didn't have much in common with them. I liked trucks better than dolls when I was little and sports better than gymnastics as I got older. I still don't like 'girly' things, and at a party you'll always find me talking about sports and politics and business with the guys, not clothes and children and gossip with the women." But things got complicated when she fell in love. "My best friend was the nicest man in the world. But I didn't have the good sense to fall in love with him," she says. "Instead, I fell hard and fast for one of his army buddies. I was in bed with the guy before I knew what was happening, and married to him within six months." To her surprise, her friend did not respond well to the match. "I'm not quite sure what happened. He was angry and wouldn't talk to me for a long time, but I kept bugging him, and finally he said that I had betrayed him. How could that be true? He wasn't my lover. We weren't even sexually attracted. So how did I betray him?"

Friendships with guys can fill gaps left by friendships with women. Eileen, who married the brother of her best friend, Liz, said, "I guess it's not really surprising that I also got close to Lizzie's husband. He and I had so much in common, starting with the fact that we were outsiders who were swooped up into this noisy, loving, and controlling Chinese family!" She laughed a little self-consciously and said, "I'm not saying anything they wouldn't tell you. They *are* controlling! He's Chinese, so he knew the customs that I didn't know; but he's quieter and less outgoing, and we helped buffer each other from the family when we needed it." Eileen and her brother-in-law also had a common interest in Chinese art. "We started a business together, supporting young Chinese artists who wanted to create classic-style paintings in the post-Communist era.

We provided them with an international market where they could sell their paintings. We're really good work partners and friends."

Even if the sexual attraction in a relationship with a guy friend is one-sided, it may exist more often than we realize.[12] It seems that even among millennials, who may be more comfortable than older generations with the idea of non-romantic sex, men are more motivated by sexual desire, even in platonic male-female friendships, while women are more often looking for emotional connection.[13] Sometimes when attraction becomes mutual, there is often an agreement, spoken or unspoken, that the friendship is more important than a sexual relationship.

Unresolved sexual tension between fictional characters keeps us coming back to some of our favorite television and book series. But in real life, these feelings can create serious problems. Numerous women told me about having to end a friendship with a guy because the sexual tension was too hard for one or the other to handle. Angelica, a wiry, high-energy divorcée, told me that she had "no patience for it. If a guy wants to be a friend, there can't be any sexual undercurrents. The nonverbal communications will drive us both crazy."

Only a few of the women I interviewed were involved in such high drama. "I go running with my husband's best friend," said one former athlete. "We've got a very close relationship of our own. A lot of times we'll go out for a quick drink or something, just to check in on each other. But it's very clear that there's nothing between us other than a close friendship." Another woman told me that her husband loved basketball and his best friend loved classical music. "So sometimes my husband will go out with the guys to a game, and his friend and I will go to a concert. It's a perfect arrangement. Everybody gets to do what they like best."

A number of women are just more at home with guys. A law student said, "I prefer what the guys have to say; but I also like being the only girl in a group. It's not that I'm flirting with the guys or anything like that. In a group of women, there's this silent competitive thing going on. You're always wondering, Who's prettier? Who's more popular? In a group of guys, well . . . there's competition, but it's friendlier."

In general researchers have found that despite our differences, men and women value similar qualities in friends. We all appreciate friends who are supportive, dependable, caring, trustworthy, and fun.[14] The popularity of rom-coms about best friends falling in love and living happily ever after notwithstanding, researchers have found that most male-female friendship dyads remain nonsexual, even when friends are physically attracted to each other.[15] From my wide-ranging discussions, it seems to me that the same can be said about friendship dyads of two women. For the most part, we seem to be pretty good at managing sexual tension, when it arises, without destroying our friendships.

When a Friend Changes Gender

Whether you are going through the transgender process or trying to connect with a friend who is, this change can pose challenges to relationships. This remains true even today, when issues of gender are discussed more freely and variations in gender expression are more widely accepted and appear in the news and popular entertainment. For instance, in *Sense8,* the Netflix sci-fi series, the trans actress Jamie Clayton portrays a transgender character named Nomi, but her gender is not meant to be a significant factor in the storyline.

Yet conflicts can emerge among friends during this transition. Annie, a recent college grad, says that she had been friendly with a guy through high school. "We went to the same college together, but he started hanging out with the LGBQT kids. I liked a bunch of them, but that wasn't my 'group.' I had other friends and other activities, and he and I sort of lost touch. Then I heard that he had a new name. I wasn't sure whether he had gone through the medical changes or not, but the next time I ran into him — her — on campus, it was clear that she was trans. I was down with it and tried to be friendly, but she didn't seem to want to have anything to do with me."

When a friend or an acquaintance changes gender, it often upsets our own sense of balance. We can also become uncomfortable with what our friend's change means about our own sense of femininity. This is what happened for Jessica, a paralegal, who had a work friend who went through a gender change. "We were friends when she was a woman, but when she made herself into a guy, she still wanted to be friends. Except I think she — he — was looking for more than a friendship. I wasn't comfortable with that at all. I mean, I had known him as a woman, and I had trouble making the transition with him. And I was kind of skived by the whole thing. I wished him all the happiness in the world, and if he needed to do it, then good for him. But I couldn't be what he wanted me to be. He finally just sort of stopped coming around."

Can Your Husband, Wife, or Life Partner Be Your Best Friend?

Many women told me that their husband, wife, or life partner was their best friend. As one fifty-five-year-old grandmother said, "I'd rather spend my time with my husband than with anyone else except my grandchildren." And an empty-nester said, "I miss my kids, but I'm really lucky, because I love spending time with my husband. We enjoy so many of the same things, and we have the same values and beliefs. We even have the same sense of humor. So the upside of having the kids gone is that I get to spend more time with my closest friend in the world."

John Helliwell, a professor and researcher at the University of Vancouver, studies happiness around the world. He and his colleague Shawn Grover found that couples who said that their best friend was also their spouse scored twice as high on a scale of life satisfaction than did other couples.[16] Helliwell and Grover hypothesize that having a sexual partner with whom you can also talk and share life struggles is an important part of feeling satisfied with your life, even in difficult times.

However, women who told me that their spouse, male or female, was their best friend also said that they worried a little about being in a cocoon with their loved one. A lively hairdresser whose husband had recently undergone surgery for prostate cancer said, "I've been thinking about what would happen if he got really sick, or if he died. I got scared and started thinking that I need to expand my circle of friends so that I'm not completely dependent on him."

A beautifully dressed executive assistant married to another woman said, "The problem for us is that we are too happy being alone together. We are totally dependent on each other for everything. I don't think it's completely healthy."

On the other hand, a single bookkeeper in her forties said, "I don't think there are any rules about this. I wish people would pay more attention to what they want, and not to what is supposed to be right." She told me that she loved her work and her single life. "I know it's kind of odd, but I really like being alone," she said, "but I also care about my friends. I have a couple of male friends who are my sexual partners, but I wouldn't want to be married to either of them. Well, I don't want to be married to anyone. I don't think I could possibly be more satisfied with my life than I am right now." Bella DePaulo, author of *Singled Out* and a *Psychology Today* blogger, says something similar. In an email to the *Huffington Post,* she writes, "For people like me who are single at heart, getting married may not have the same implications as it does for the kinds of people who want to marry and choose to do so."[17]

One fifty-two-year-old phlebotomist, though, saw definite benefits to her marriage, and specifically to her marriage to a woman. "We talk about everything," she said. Research has shown that talking is one of the keys to keeping a relationship in balance.[18] And we women are famous for our capacity to talk about things.

Melody told me that she thought this was why she and her childhood best friend were able to find a good balance. "It wasn't that we always wanted exactly the same thing from our friendship," she said. "But we were able to talk about everything, so we didn't let anything get out of control. When we roomed together after college, we had to talk about stupid things, like somebody's hair always in the bathtub drain, or gross things like used sanitary napkins that weren't thrown away, or dirty dishes and overflowing ashtrays. And boyfriends. And parents. We know everything there is to know about each other, and we've talked about it. So it's not a big deal to say that we're turned on by each other, or that we love each other, or that we hate each other in a given moment, for a given reason."

But talking about everything does not come easily to everyone, even women. Some studies have shown that at least some of the traditional imbalance between genders may have less to do with whether a person is a man or a woman, and more to do with who has more or less power.[19] Women's friendships are often based on a sense of equality, which can involve complementarity or a meshing of roles, rather than an exactly even balance.[20]

"We are part of a large circle of friends, but my wife is my best friend, my soulmate, and my sexual partner," said one woman. "And that's how I want it to be."

But what happens when the balance is off kilter?

Several women told me that they had broken up with a romantic partner who had difficulty sharing her affection and time. One working mom in her forties said, "My partner is a good mother to our children, but she can't stand that I focus a lot of my extra time on the children. I work long hours, and when I get home, I want to know how they're doing. I want some cuddle time with them. But she has been with them all day and she wants cuddle time from me. We fight a lot because she says I'm not available enough to her. We used to be best friends as well as lovers and life partners. Now I feel like I have to get my friendship needs met outside of our relationship. It makes me very sad. It's not what I want, but I don't know how to fix it."

What You Can Do

Sometimes talking about things is the best solution, even when it feels like the hardest. But talking is not, as we now know, always easy, and at times it doesn't even help. Many women find that their guy friends are happy "just to let things be," as one recent college grad put it. "I have a great friend who I mainly see at the gym," she said. "We're workout partners, and we chat about everything all through our workouts. He has a girlfriend, and he talks about her a lot, so I know there's nothing romantic there. But I felt the need just to put it into words. I don't know why, but I think I was worried that he might think I was more interested in him as a potential boyfriend, so I said something like, 'You know we're just friends, right?' and he looked at me like I had grown another head. I laughed it off, and things went back to normal. But I learned my lesson! Don't talk about things you don't need to talk about with a guy friend!"

But sometimes talking does help. For example, the Israeli accountant who married her best friend's best friend says that talking saved the friendship. "I told him that I loved him and always would love him," she told me. "And I said that I didn't want to lose our friendship, so he needed to talk to me about what was going on. I couldn't fall out of love with his best friend, but I could show how important he was to me. The good news was that he was also important to my husband, so I made both of them keep talking about it, with me and with each other. We all muddled our way through till we got to a much better place."

The same, of course, is true with our women friends. Sexual feelings are extremely difficult to talk about, and sometimes it is better to leave some things unsaid. But talking can also ease a complicated situation. Interestingly, it is not always necessary to address the feelings directly. The psychologist who managed to work things out with her friend who wanted a romantic relationship says, "We did talk, but very briefly. I took my courage in my hands and told her that I thought she was coming on to me, and that I wasn't going to be able to respond. And I said I loved her and didn't want to lose her as a friend, so what could we do about it? Her answer was kind of amazing. She said, 'Okay, I needed to know that. Let me deal with it for a while, and then we'll be all right.' And that's exactly what happened. I gave her space to deal with it, and we moved on. Together."

Research has shown that close relationships affect our sense of well-being. The psychologist Matthew Lieberman tells us that our brains are wired to connect.[21] Attachment theorists and neuroscientists like Allan Schore and Daniel Siegel agree.[22] But as Deborah Tannen points out, there are many different ways of connecting.[23] What is important, say Nicholas Christakis and James Fowler, authors of *Connected,* is to understand that our own varied and individual ways of connecting are key to our emotional and physical well-being.[24] So it may just be that how and with whom you connect is less important than *that* you connect.

10

~

Do Good Boundaries Make Bad Friends?

EVA WAS IN HER MID-THIRTIES AND PREGNANT WITH her second child when her best friend, Helena, hit a painful time in her own life. "She was involved with a man who didn't want to get married and didn't want to have children. She would come over and hang out with me, but she didn't want to play with my four-year-old or do anything except talk about her relationship." Eva felt guilty about not being responsive to Helena. "I know what it's like. I've been there, when all I can think about is my own pain. But I hope, although maybe I'm wrong, that I'm never so completely self-centered that I don't pay attention to anyone else's needs."

Torn between her desire to be a good friend who could respond to what Helena so clearly needed from her and her equally strong desire to be available to her son, Eva gradually found herself resenting her friend. "I just wasn't going to plop him down in front of the television for two or three hours while she told me how unhappy she was. But she didn't understand. All she could see was how much she needed me. After a while, I stopped feeling sympathetic, and I stopped being available so much when she asked if she could come over to talk. But I felt so guilty. Helena was my best friend, and I cared deeply for her. I felt like the worst friend in the world."

Research has shown that marriage and child rearing often alter the kinds of friends we have.[1] In part, these changes happen because we no longer have the time for the intense physical and emotional intimacy of college friendships, with middle-of-the-night conversations over ice cream and popcorn. As we get older, we have different goals and needs, and we sometimes feel as if we become different people as we go through the developmental phases of adulthood. As one twenty-six-year-old told me, "Your body changes. You fill out in funny places. And your psyche changes too. You become a woman physically and emotionally. You just don't feel so merged with your girlfriends anymore. You have different interests, even if you still care a lot about each other." This young woman was not married, but she was working long hours at an exciting career. "I love my friends," she said. "But some of them don't understand why I'm not available the way I used to be. If they don't get it, then I'm sad about it, but I can't stay friends with them. I just don't have that in me anymore."

Erin, a twenty-three-year-old with big brown eyes magnified by thick glasses, said, "I sometimes forget about my friends. I mean, I forget to get back to them after they've sent me a message or something." She said that sometimes she got tied up in a work assignment or in an activity with other friends, and the response slipped her mind. "But other times, maybe I don't really want to do what they're asking me about, or there's some other reason I don't want to keep the thread going. So it just goes out of my head." She told me that she often felt that this made her a bad friend. "But a lot of my friends just ignore it. They sort of seem to accept that it's just who I am. 'Oh, Erin, she's such an airhead,' is how they deal with it. They don't take it personally. But I don't think it's a very good way for a friend to behave. I'm trying to be better about it."

Like many other women I spoke with, Erin told me that she sometimes has trouble being direct with her friends. "Like, when I just don't want to do something, I have trouble saying it." Not responding is a way of responding, though. Erin added, "But I guess the point gets across."

Other women also said that they had difficulty saying no even to their closest friends. "I don't want to hurt anyone's feelings," said one busy saleswoman. "So I end up doing things I don't want to do, or I just don't respond. Either way I feel lousy about myself. I want to learn to be more direct, but I don't want to be a bad friend. How can you be a good friend and say no? That's something I haven't figured out."

Setting Boundaries

A young lawyer had just been hired for the job of her dreams in a firm that provided free legal assistance to people who could not afford to pay. The work was exciting but also demanding, and she was worn out by the time she got home each night. She said, "I was talking to an old friend, who is extremely empathetic. Whatever the person she's talking to is going through, she wholeheartedly takes on that experience herself. It's like she is also going through it with them. She is very supportive and generous with her time. She will go to your house or for coffee or lunch with you, even if it's at a time that's completely inconvenient for her. But I don't have time to be that kind of friend. And even if I did have the time, that's not who I am. I'm not at all giving and generous like she is. I guess that makes me a bad friend."

Another woman talked about her sympathy for a friend who wanted more of her time and attention after they were both married. "She somehow thought we would still be joined at the hip, the way we were before we got married. I understood how much she wanted that connection with me, and I knew she didn't understand what had happened to it. Well, to tell you the truth, I don't think I knew, either. But I just wasn't interested in being so close anymore. I felt terrible about not responding to her needs. It was selfish of me, I know. But I felt like I had to live my life. We stopped being friends. Nothing was ever said, but it just didn't work. I've always felt bad about that."

This discomfort with not being available enough for a friend bothers many women. But what is enough, anyway? Like the young lawyer and the new bride, many women feel that being a good friend means being boundlessly available and giving.

Yet it is not always possible to give selflessly and also take care of your own needs. It is also not even the best way to be a good friend. At thirty-six, Nila was part of a group of women who had been together since first grade. "We've been through every part of life together. We've weathered boyfriends, marriages and divorces, pregnancy, miscarriages, childbirth, and the death of one child. Husbands have gotten ill, and one of us has had breast cancer. We've supported each other through all of these things, and through serious problems with our parents and siblings — in fact, those problems are some of the things that we bonded over when we were young."

She says that the group members have learned that "no one can be there for you all the time. Sometimes your feelings might be hurt if one of the women doesn't call to check in on you when you're having a hard time. Or, we have a group email going, and sometimes one person gets off the list for a period of time. The first time it happened we were all a little upset. But we talked about it, and we realized that we need to have space from each other sometimes."

Many women think that boundaries and empathy are opposites, and that good friends have limitless empathy for one another. But is unlimited empathy really the core of women's friendships? To answer that question, we need to look first at what we mean by these terms.

According to *The American Heritage Dictionary,* a boundary is "something that indicates a border or limit."[2] Emotional limits are often subtle or vague, so recognizing them can be difficult. Interestingly, empathy, or "the ability to identify with or understand the perspective, experiences, or motivations of another individual and to comprehend and share another individual's emotional state," can help us recognize, set, and respect healthy boundaries.[3]

In her book *The Gifts of Imperfection: Let Go of Who You Think You're Supposed to Be and Embrace Who You Are,* Brené Brown writes, "When we fail to set boundaries and hold people accountable, we feel used and mistreated. This is why we sometimes attack who they are, which is far more hurtful than addressing a behavior or a choice."[4] Nila, like many of the women who told me of long-term, successful friendships, said, "I think the key to our relationships is honesty — brutal honesty sometimes. We tell each other when our feelings are hurt. And we call each other out on behaviors that are totally selfish or self-serving. Like, we have one friend who is always late to everything. She can really screw up plans, say, if we've got tickets to a movie or a concert. So we've told her that it really bothers us, and we don't let her off the hook. But we also have figured out ways to deal with it. We give her her own ticket, so she can arrive when she can. I mean, we're not going to change her. So we sort of make it into a joke, and we tease her, and we also let her know that we miss her when she's not there. And we tell her directly when it upsets us that she's late to something really important, like a baby-naming."

In other words, Nila and her women friends have found ways to set clear boundaries while also maintaining caring, empathic relationships.

Boundaries protect our friendships. As one stay-at-home mom put it, "I'm trying to teach my children to have respect for each other's personal and physical space. I grew up in a house where there was no such thing as a closed door and no respect for privacy. There was a positive side to it. My mom never turned a friend away. Everyone knew they could come to her with any problem, anytime. But there was a negative side too. Our house was always chaotic. Nothing ever got finished. And Mom never had time for herself. She was a talented artist, but she was so busy taking care of us kids and everybody else in her life that she never fulfilled her own talent. Even after we were all grown up, she was always too busy doing things for other people to spend time doing something that would have given her great pleasure. I think she always felt sad about it, but she didn't have the ability to say no to anyone. And she suffered a lot as a result."

Intimacy does not mean giving up your self, although cultural and psychological expectations sometimes seem to indicate that women are not supposed to have a self separate from the people we love, including our friends.[5] Often, though, when we even think about setting boundaries with a friend, we fear that it means that we are being selfish and therefore unfeminine. This is how it was for Kaisha, a tall, slim African American physician in her thirties. She said, "I know I'm feminine in some ways, like how I look, but I'm in a male-dominated field, and I have a lot of male traits. Like, for example, I prefer structure to fluidity. I'm never late, and I hate it when women friends are — and they are a lot. So I have to make a big deal about it, because I get so irritated, and then my friends give me a hard time about being too rigid — like a guy."

You, like many women, may value mutuality, equality, and complementarity in your friendships. But how do you find a good balance between your needs and those of your friends? "I don't always think my friends' needs are valid, or that they supersede mine," said Kaisha. "But when I get bored with somebody's complaints or tired of their breaking a date with me to go out with a guy, I feel like I'm not being a good friend."

Nan, a busy administrator in an architectural firm, set clear limits around her friendships. "I have work friends," she said. "And I have friends at church. But I don't have those kinds of friends who will call to talk about their personal difficulties. I never had time for that, and the truth is, I never wanted it. What do I know about psychology? I would just tell someone to see a therapist, and I don't think that's what the person wants to hear. I've always felt like there was something a little wrong with me because I didn't have those kinds of friends and didn't want them. I never said that out loud before!"

A waitress told me, "I work long hours and I'm tired of smiling and being friendly and outgoing by the time I get home. So I maintain very old-fashioned calling hours with my friends. They can call me between certain hours, and that's it. Otherwise text or email me and I'll get back to you, but not necessarily right away. I'm not spontaneous. My time is precious to me. I am also a kind and generous friend, and I have wonderful girlfriends who I love to see and spend time with. I don't have any trouble setting boundaries, because I know that I would be a terrible friend if I didn't protect my precious alone time."

Sometimes setting boundaries can feel mean and uncaring. In many of the examples I heard, what felt "mean" was simply that a woman had met her own needs instead of a friend's, and the friend's feelings had been hurt as a result. The intention was not to be unkind. However, some women told me about times they had intentionally done something hurtful to a friend. I was surprised at how often these mean behaviors could be unpacked to reveal an effort, albeit not always a well-thought-out one, to set limits or create boundaries.

We often feel guilty when we feel we are being selfish. "It doesn't seem right to ignore someone else's needs just to get what you want," said one woman in her late twenties. Yet not setting limits can also be problematic. "If you get angry because you're giving, giving, giving, and never getting back, then that's not any good either," said another twenty-something. Difficulties with boundaries are often directly related to the need to please and the desire to be connected. You might worry that no matter how nicely you say no, a friend might get angry and end the relationship. And of course, sometimes this does happen. You might also wish that you could be more like your mother or grandmother. An office manager in a navy blue suit and silk blouse said that she wished she had an "open heart" like her grandmother's. "That woman would welcome anyone into her home, day or night. Friends often came over to her house to get a little TLC — and a piece of her incredible pie that was always waiting for takers. I'm not like that. I wish I was."

Psychoanalysts have had a field day with the idea of guilt, or the feeling that you have done something wrong. For women, these feelings are often related to a need to please others and also to cultural expectations that link femininity to kindness, nurturing, and selflessness.[6] On his *Psychology Today* blog, the psychologist Guy Winch[7] tells us that guilt can play an important role in friendships, since it signals to us that we have done or are about to do something that could be hurtful to another person. We can then either avoid the behavior or take action to deal with the consequences. But for women, the signals that guilt sends to our psyches can be misleading.

Nila and her friends, for instance, would never have been able to maintain their close bonds if they had felt guilty about setting limits with one another. "All of us have friends outside the group as well. We might have had some problems if we felt guilty about having those other connections. But we are all aware that we can't meet every need for every one of us. We're like a family. We're there, and we'll always be there. But you also need other connections, outside the family. And sometimes that means you have to say no to something that the group wants to do because you're busy with your other friends. We deal with it. Nobody needs to feel guilty about it."

A number of women also spoke of helping to nurse friends through illnesses. Each of them struggled with pain and guilt about not doing enough, despite knowing, at least intellectually, that they had done as much as anyone could.

What You Can Do

Sometimes guilt has underlying meaning. It can be helpful, although not always easy, to understand what else our psyche might be trying to communicate to us with this feeling.

Attachment, feminist, and relational theorists say that women often fear confrontation because connections are so important to us, and we worry that open disagreement will lead to anger and disconnection.[8] Avoiding boundaries can be a way of protecting yourself from both anger and loss. But, as we have seen, sometimes we lose a friendship precisely because we did not openly confront a difficulty or set boundaries to make the relationship manageable.

If your friend needs to talk to you in the middle of the night, the way she did when you were in college, but you need to get a good night's sleep because you have an important meeting at work the next day, you might decide that her needs outweigh your own, particularly if she is in crisis, or if it is a once-in-a-great-while request. But in a balanced, mutual friendship, she will also respect your need to be well rested the next day and will try not to keep you on the phone too long. Of course, that can happen only if you let her know that you have the presentation and would like to get to sleep, which is setting a boundary. You can set boundaries simply and gently, but you also might want to practice being direct. As the author Megan LeBoutillier puts it, "'No' is a complete sentence."[9]

Kaisha liked the idea that her need for structure was as valid as a friend's need to complain. "I guess, if it's really balanced and mutual, then things would even out if sometimes I would tolerate her complaints and sometimes she would make sure to get to a date with me on time!"

In a friendship characterized by balance and mutuality, your friend will not call you every night at midnight because she cannot get to sleep because she understands that you go to sleep earlier than she does. But when a friend does not respect your needs, what do you do?

A massage therapist in her forties told me that she had learned about the importance of setting boundaries in her work. "Massage is an intimate experience, and people are vulnerable when they're in your space. A lot of times clients will talk to me like I'm their therapist. I have to be careful to help them feel safe with me, which means protecting their boundaries and maintaining mine as well. I don't share all of my personal life with clients, and I don't talk about what they say to me to anyone else. And when someone asks me for an appointment at a time that doesn't work for me, I'm fine with saying that I can't do it. But when it comes to friends and family, I have a much harder time.

"I had a friend who always called at nine o'clock at night. She would talk on and on about her day, her life, whatever. She wasn't just talking about herself, though; she wanted to know how I was doing too. But I didn't want to talk. It's a bad time for me. I'm usually exhausted, and I just want to put my feet up and watch some mindless television for a half hour. I couldn't tell her. I felt like it was selfish of me not to give her that little bit of time. But I sort of resented her. It's not fair, because I didn't tell her why I didn't want to talk."

The problem was not selfishness, but an unwillingness to set limits that would protect the friendship in the long run. We are not all capable of, or even interested in, practicing the kind of honesty that Nila and her friends achieved, but their ability to do so can serve as a powerful reminder that setting limits does not have to destroy a friendship. In fact, sometimes those limits are precisely what make deep and meaningful friendship possible. So when you worry that you are not being a good enough friend, ask yourself these questions:

Did I do something mean or did I set a boundary that my friend did not like, but that I needed for myself?

If I did something that hurt my friend's feelings, even unintentionally, can I apologize for what I did and move on?

Is there some other feeling or concern underlying my guilt that I need to deal with?

If you can answer "yes" to any or all of these questions, you might be able to let yourself off the hook. If you are not sure about the answers or feel that you in fact did do something wrong, you, like many other women, may need help dealing with anger and conflict in your friendships. And that's what we will explore next.

11

~

Why Do Women Friends Hold Grudges Forever?

MANAGING ANGER, JUDGMENT, AND SHAME

NEVER GET ANGRY AT MY FRIENDS," LILIANA, A TALL, dark-haired woman in her thirties, told me. "Sometimes I'm disappointed in them, but things always blow over. It's not a problem."

"I used to have a friend who remembered every mistake you ever made," said a hairdresser with pink highlights in her black hair. "I stopped being friends with her. She just wasn't good for me."

"Women don't blow up at each other unless something really, really bad happens. We keep it all inside, but then when there's an explosion, it's really hard to repair the damage," said a busy stay-at-home mother.

"One of the reasons I prefer to be friends with men," said one businesswoman, "is that they let go of their anger so much more easily than women do. A guy gets angry, he lets you know, and then he moves on. A woman gets angry, she doesn't tell you, and she holds a grudge against you forever."

These sentiments were repeated in a variety of ways by many of the women I talked with, but they are also reflected in recent research. A study done at Harvard University, for example, found that women stayed angry and held grudges longer than men.[1] The researchers found that after a disagreement, men were friendlier and more likely to physically connect with one another — with a handshake or a hug — than were women. In popular shows about women's friendships, arguments frequently either go underground or end the relationship. One reason for the international popularity of the various Real Housewives series could very well be the regularity with which the women on the shows get into outraged — and frequently outrageous — name-calling and friendship-ending, something we find it difficult to do in the real world.

What makes it so hard for us to fight openly and honestly with our women friends and then make up and move on?

The Harvard researchers suggest that men forgive and forget more quickly than women do because of evolution. In the days when men had to hunt together to find food or band together to protect their tribes, they had to work together, which meant finding ways to resolve conflict and let go of discord relatively quickly. Women, on the other hand, were more focused on protecting their homes and their children. They therefore benefited from remembering past aggression because it helped them stay prepared for the next danger.

Whether or not this reasoning makes sense or fits with what we see in the world, it does seem that we women often have trouble expressing anger on the one hand, and forgiving our friends' transgressions on the other. Yet at the same time, students of female psychology say that we are quick to compromise and to let go of our own position, even our own point of view, sometimes to our own detriment. One problem, as Cathi Hanauer tells us, is that anger often has multiple causes.[2]

Fear of Retaliation

Many women hide angry feelings from friends because they fear that the friends will retaliate in the form of angry recriminations, name-calling, or hurtful attacks. We also fear that a friend will say bad things about us, tell other people things we've said in confidence, or post negative or even hateful information on social media. No wonder we avoid angry confrontations. But for many women, the possibility of withdrawal, when a friend simply stops being a friend, feels even more threatening. As we know, for some of us, maintaining connections is sometimes more important than anything else. So the fear that a friend might stop talking to you, remove your number from her phone, or unfriend you on Facebook or otherwise disconnect from you on social media can outweigh your anger, irritation, or frustration and keep you quiet.

For example, the psychologist Jeanne Safer became frustrated with a dear friend who had become increasingly self-involved. This friend talked on and on about herself and her problems without ever asking about Dr. Safer, who writes that even though "I prided myself on addressing problems in relationships, I never felt I could reveal my growing discontent without risking her displeasure."[3] Dr. Safer hesitated because of her friend's short temper.

Some of the women I spoke with told me they avoided confronting friends because they did not like loud arguments, and many said something similar to this: they were afraid of displeasing friends with whom they felt angry. Some were afraid of heated confrontations, while others worried that a friend would talk about them behind their back. "It's that old thing about being ostracized by the 'in-group,' left over from middle school," said one thirty-two-year-old.

Others were concerned about how they would sound and look while confronting a friend. "I'm embarrassed to bring it up," said a twenty-four-year-old about her irritation with a roommate who kept leaving dirty dishes in the kitchen sink. "It makes me sound so dumb. And what if she starts telling me about all the things she doesn't like about me. It's not worth it to me."

The psychologist Harriet Lerner says that we worry that our anger will turn everyone off."[4] Many of the women I spoke with told me that along with shame about their angry feelings, they were afraid that friends would dislike them and reject them if they openly expressed anger. Interestingly, the only situation in which it seems to be okay to do so is when our anger is not about our own needs but serves to protect someone else. For example, for a long time Paula, on *Crazy Ex-Girlfriend,* supports her best friend Rebecca in her crazy pursuit of her non-boyfriend Josh. When Rebecca is unkind to her, Paula just sucks it up because it seems that best friends aren't allowed to be angry at each other. But ultimately she blasts Rebecca for being self-destructive, and this time her expression of anger seems fine — even good — because it comes from her desire to take care of Rebecca.

Ashamed to Be Angry

Even when justified, however, direct anger can evoke shame and embarrassment for many women. When we get angry with a friend, we may worry that we are not being a good friend or even a good woman, which leads to shame. In her popular TED Talk and her book *Daring Greatly,* the author Brené Brown tells us that shame can be a straitjacket for many women. Shame, or a sense of humiliation about doing something wrong, can keep us from clearing the air.

This is how it worked for Yvonne, a physician who had been part of a close-knit group since high school. "I once tried to fix up one of the girls with a guy from the hospital where I work," she told me. "They were both telling me about being lonely, and I thought they would get along well. But it turned out that the guy was trying to hit on me, and I hadn't realized it. He told my friend that I was 'hot' and asked if she thought I would ever go out with him. My friend didn't speak to me for a year after that. She said I had done it on purpose, and wouldn't listen to anything I said. I didn't do it on purpose, I wouldn't do anything like that, but I was hurt that she would think that I would."

It is possible that Yvonne's friend was as hurt and humiliated by the fact that this guy had not been interested in her as she was by Yvonne's supposed trickery. Like Yvonne, she may have been too uncomfortable to acknowledge what she was feeling, so shame may have kept them from communicating and clearing the air. Yvonne said, "It made the group really uncomfortable for all of us for a while. I had to stay away from things that she was going to be part of. It wasn't fair, but it was the only way to manage the situation that I could figure out."

Tina, a yoga teacher in her early thirties, painted a picture of anger in a way I heard many times. "When I was in my twenties, my parents, whose marriage had always been awful, went through a terrible divorce. I was angry all of the time, but nobody under-stood, because I was supposed to be an adult, and they thought it shouldn't matter to me that my parents couldn't stand each other. I got into some kind of argument with my roommate, who was my best friend, about something that wasn't even important — maybe her not picking up her wet towel and hanging it on the towel rack after her shower. I'm a bit of a neat freak, so it was probably some-thing like that. She told me that she couldn't stand to be around me anymore, because I was a crazy woman. I'm not sure that I understood, even then, that I was angry. I was just hurting so much inside. But it was destroying my relationships. I figured out that I needed to get a handle on this stuff before I lost all of my friends."

Tina put her finger on a difficulty we often have about telling friends when we are angry with them: some of the *reasons* that we get angry make us uncomfortable. We worry that our friend will think we are being petty, mean, or silly, which makes it hard to talk about the thing that is bothering us. A professional office cleaner told me that she was friendly with a group of women who had all grown up in the same community. "One of the girls is a real people magnet. She stays in touch with everyone. But I don't like her. I don't trust her. Can't really tell you why, except that she's kind of manipulative. I haven't ever told this to anyone else. But sometimes she leaves me out of some of the plans on purpose. She just doesn't let me know what's happening. It hurts my feelings and it makes me mad, but I know what she's doing. I think my other friends will say I'm being paranoid, so I don't say anything to anybody. I just try to ignore her and go around her, making my plans without her interference."

Another woman told me, "It's hard to talk to a friend about something she's doing that bothers you when you feel embarrassed about being bothered by it. Like, I hate the sound of people chewing with their mouth open, and one of my girlfriends chews with her mouth open all the time. I once asked her to stop, and she told me I was crazy, she wasn't doing that. So now I don't say anything about it to her because I know she'll look at me like I'm nuts. I just have to try to make sure I don't sit near her when we're eating, because it really makes me so mad when she smacks her food."

Many women told me that they did not like to express their anger because it made them look bad. "I don't want people to think of me as that crazy woman who goes off her nutter all the time," said one generally outspoken woman. Another said, "It's not a pretty sight, when a woman gets really enraged. I don't want to be like that." And yet another told me, "I have memories of my mom losing it when I was a kid. Her eyes got really crazy. I don't want to ever be like her."

Anger as a Signal

Because we fear that anger will be disruptive, we avoid it, send it underground, or direct it at a target that cannot reject us, like a child, a pet, a family member, or ourselves. Yet such redirection can create problems in other relationships that you value, damage your self-esteem, and even, when buried or turned on yourself, potentially lead to health issues such as headaches, digestive problems, insomnia, anxiety, depression, and skin problems.[5] The answer is not to go around blasting everyone you are angry at, but to find healthy ways to process the feelings. Talking about the feelings and resolving conflict is one way to manage these emotions, but it is not always the best solution — and it is not always possible.

Before deciding whether or not to talk to a friend about something she did or didn't do that upset you, it can be helpful to keep in mind that angry feelings serve an important purpose. Harriet Lerner tells us, "Anger is a signal, and one worth listening to."[6] According to Heinz Kohut, the originator of self psychology, anger is frequently a sign that we are feeling hurt, powerless, or frightened. But because we often shove anger aside before determining what it is signaling, many women have difficulties deciphering the message that their psyche is sending. Sometimes friends can help us figure out what the feelings mean and how to process them.

This is how it worked for Yvonne, who thought she was doing her friend a favor by fixing her up with a colleague. She said that the group finally told the two women "that we needed to stop behaving like children. They said they understood that we were both hurt and upset, but that we had to talk about what had happened so we could move on." Each of them got a chance to explain her side of the story and her feelings about the incident. "We both got our feelings out, and we each said that we had not meant to hurt the other. And then, of course, we cried, and everybody cried, and we hugged each other. And truly surprising, to me at least — that was the end of it."

Many women told me that they had been able to stay friends with other women throughout their lives because they could talk to them about anything. As one mother who was still close to a group of women from elementary school put it, "Brutal honesty has kept us together. We know each other really, really well. The good stuff, of course, which is the glue that keeps us connected. But we know each other's dirty laundry too. We don't ever throw it in anybody's face, but we do keep each other honest. Sometimes we do it gently, or with humor or a little bit of teasing. But when one woman in the group started flirting too hard with another one's husband, we all called her on it. It just wasn't going to work. We told her that we valued our friendships more than anything, and she was going to destroy something really meaningful with a stupid flirtation. She was upset and angry, and she said that she wasn't breaking up a happy marriage, that our other friend needed to take an honest look at her marriage. It was painful all around, but both of the women eventually acknowledged that it had been an important wake-up call to get their lives back on track."

Managing Conflict

The authors of the book *Difficult Conversations: How to Discuss What Matters Most*[7] tell us that we often leave out some of the most important thoughts and feelings when we are trying to resolve conflict. Because so many women carry an image of friendship that looks like that ideal match — two friends who understand everything about each other without words — talking about dissimilarities doesn't come easily. Many women told me that they had difficulties factoring difference into their friendships. Liz, who had been best friends with Eileen from the age of twelve, echoed something I heard repeatedly. "I had troubles when I realized that Eileen wasn't my exact clone. It made me angry that she didn't see things the same way that I did. I didn't know how to handle it, so I stopped talking to her for a while."

The need for a friend to be an exact replica of our own self, however, seems to shift as we get older. Liz and Eileen both told me that they had discovered that their differences added richness to their relationship. "I can still understand how Lizzie is feeling," said Eileen, "and she understands me. But we know now that we have to find ways to talk about some things in order to deepen that sort of mutuality. And sometimes when we do, we also learn something new about ourselves." She stops for a minute, then adds, "Or about our children. I have a daughter who is so much like Lizzie, it's scary. When she says something I don't get, I channel Lizzie in my head, and nine times out of ten, I can figure out what's going on with my daughter."

A homemaker in her sixties told me that when she was younger, most of her friends had been very much like her, with the same values, religious practices, and politics. But as she got older, she began to change some of her own opinions. "I'm not so religious anymore, for example. And my politics are different, so I don't always agree with some of the things my old friends say. But it's a lot easier to talk to some of my new friends about our differences than to try to explain them to people I've known for a long time." Like many women I spoke with, as she got older, she felt more comfortable expressing her own opinions, but she realized that she had to choose when to argue and when to keep quiet. "It's interesting to me. I don't worry so much about people getting angry with me these days. I think that's a function of my age, to tell you the truth. But with some of my oldest friends, who don't understand this change in me, I try not to get into political discussions. When the issues do come up, I try to tactfully change the subject. And when that doesn't work, I just gently say, 'I don't think we want to go there, do you?' Most of the time that's enough to get them to change direction. Because an argument with them would go nowhere, and feelings would probably get hurt."

Many women agreed that it's important to know when *not* to talk things out. In Sue Grafton's novel *X*, the narrator and private investigator Kinsey Millhone has an argument with her friend Ruthie about some damning information that has surfaced about Ruthie's idealized and recently deceased husband. With Ruthie giving her the silent treatment, Kinsey wonders whether she should ignore the problem or try to force her friend to talk more about it. She decides, "The practice of baring all, analyzing every nuance embedded in a quarrel, is a surefire way to keep an argument alive. Better to establish a temporary peace and revisit the conflict later."[8] She says that after a cooling-off period, the issue that started the disagreement often feels far less important than the friendship itself.

Sometimes not talking about a problem is the best thing you can do for your friendship. A thirty-year-old who told me that she made friends easily and kept them "forever" said, "Sometimes staying friends is more important than winning an argument." The important thing is to know that you have a choice, and that you can make a decision about whether or not to discuss an issue. But not all friends give you an option.

Grudge-Holding and Grudge-Holders

Sometimes a friend seems to need to hold on to a grudge. "I had a best friend who could never let anyone off the hook," said one woman. "If you said or did something that upset her, she just stopped talking to you. And she never spoke to you again. So of course I worried about doing something that would set her off. I never did, but I watched myself closely. I don't think it was good for the friendship in the long run."

Grudge-holding is often closely tied to feelings of victimization or martyrdom; in these cases we hold on to a sense of having been wronged, even in the face of apologies and attempts to make things right. The clinical social worker, psychotherapist, and minister Nancy Colier says a grudge is also a way of establishing an identity as "someone who has been wronged."[9] It can also be a way of getting sympathy from others.

A grudge-holder communicates, "I am a good and innocent person, and you have done something to distress me. Therefore, you are a bad person." On the surface, grudges help protect self-esteem; a grudge-holder gets to see herself as the "good" one. In psychotherapy, as we have seen, this is called "splitting" — all of the positive qualities are assigned to one person and all of the bad to another. Women sometimes maintain the position of innocent victim, someone with the right to be angry and to punish the person who injured her. Holding this attitude is the only way that these women feel comfortable expressing anger. The grudge-holder feels that her anger is justified, so she continues to feel good about herself.

There are several problems with this position. One, of course, is that most of us are a combination of so-called good and bad qualities, and psychological and emotional health requires that we find some way to integrate these different parts of ourselves into a basically positive sense of who we are. Another is that this kind of splitting can leave a friendship in tatters. Another difficulty occurs when a grudge and the anger that accompanies it are disproportionate to the "wrong" — for instance, when an event triggers old resentments that may have nothing to do with the incident or even the friendship itself. A dog walker in her thirties told me, "My best friend once teased me about loving dogs more than people. She didn't mean anything by it, but it touched a painful chord for me. I've always felt like there was something wrong with me because what she said is true. I've really worked at being friends with her, and I thought she understood how sensitive I was to the subject. I couldn't tell her how much she had hurt me. I just had to stop talking to her for a while. She didn't understand, and I know I hurt her, but I was too angry to tell her what was going on. I was afraid of what I would say. It took me a long time to get over it, and when I finally did, I could tell that something had changed in our friendship. It was never the same after that."

Psychologically, someone may be punishing you not only for something you actually did in the here and now, but also for a wrong or series of wrongs that the person experienced in the past. Often those wrongs happened in childhood, when the injured person had little or no power to respond. People in such situations sometimes become bitter because they had no choice but to hold the anger and resentment inside. Now they feel self-righteous about expressing those feelings — even though in truth they may be directing their hostility toward the wrong target.

What You Can Do

There is no perfect way to handle conflict with a friend. Whether you decide to open up a discussion or, like Kinsey Millhone, ride out the storm in silence, simply owning up to the fact that you are both angry can make a big difference in whether a friendship dies on the vine or gets stronger and richer.

It is important to recognize anger for what it is: a signal that often signifies the existence of other emotions that your psyche is trying to communicate to you. When anger emerges in a friendship, it often signals hurt, damaged self-esteem, feelings of powerlessness, or a sense that healthy boundaries have been broken. Because it can be hard to sort out these feelings on our own, we often turn to other friends to help us process them.

There's a danger here — the temptation to engage in malicious gossip that can further damage the conflicted friendship. If you find yourself longing to do just that, you might ask yourself if you are trying to express your own anger indirectly. Are you presenting yourself as an innocent victim and your friend as a malicious bad guy?

In the best of circumstances, your friends can help you remember that both parties in a conflict are good people. Recognizing that good people can act badly is an important part of dealing with anger. It is also part of the process of becoming a whole, emotionally healthy person. Addressing conflict can deepen and enrich a friendship. Gail Caldwell, whose memoir of her friendship with the author Caroline Knapp is a rich description of the deep connection between two women, describes such a moment.

> I blurted out, "I have to ask you something difficult — I need to know what you think of my work."
>
> She looked at me aghast. "Oh my God," she said. "I've turned into my mother. I assumed you knew how I felt, but I never told you." She rushed to reassure me, and we talked for the rest of the walk about what a swampland this was: the world of envy and rivalry and self-doubt (between women . . .)."[10]

Whether or not you decide to talk about your feelings with your friend is a matter of choice. Sometimes the healthiest position you can take is to realize that you cannot forgive a friend for something she has done. In most cases, that means letting the friendship die, although a few women I spoke with told me about managing to keep a friendship alive despite a painful wound. A forty-three-year-old store manager told me that her best friend had damaged their relationship forever by asking another woman to be her baby's godmother. "She hurt me badly, and I don't think I'll ever forgive her for it," she said, "but I still love her and care about her, and I know that she cares about me. So we will always be friends, but now with some limitations."

On the other hand, you might be pleasantly surprised if you try speaking openly to a friend about your angry feelings, especially if you can keep in mind the idea that good people can do bad things, and that friends who you love dearly can upset you. Eileen, for instance, says that talking about anger is one of the most important lessons she learned from her longtime friend Liz. "In my family, nobody says they're angry," she says. "So I was blown away the first time Lizzie told me she was mad at me. I was ready to walk away from the friendship, but to her, it was just part of being connected. When I got angry at her, I don't even remember what it was about anymore, she made me talk about it. She said that friends don't abandon each other when they're angry. They talk. I can't tell you what an impact that made on me. I think it changed my life, to tell you the truth."

In her best-selling book *The Dance of Anger,* Harriet Lerner tells us that women often learn to deny, even to themselves, that their anger exists, and because of this they keep it to themselves. When we express anger, we often do so in a less-than-productive way that leaves us feeling helpless, powerless, and self-critical. Dr. Lerner points out that anger is a signal that deserves our attention. Psychoanalysts teach us that paying attention to and respecting all of our emotions allows us to understand nonverbal messages that we are communicating to ourselves. Once you have acknowledged your anger to yourself, you have an opportunity to understand what it means. Does your anger with your friend reflect that you are feeling hurt by her, for example? Or, digging a little deeper, does it reflect guilt on your part, a fear that you have done something wrong that you are afraid to acknowledge? Women often hold grudges "forever" as a way of avoiding further pain. But in many cases, the pain comes from not allowing themselves to explore some of the different meanings that anger contains. Hurt and anger are both normal human emotions that are inevitably woven into most of our friendships, to one degree or another. There is no single right way to deal with these feelings. How you and a friend manage them will depend on the specific situation and your individual personalities. But each time you allow yourself to notice and integrate these feelings into your emotional world, you will strengthen the "feeling muscles" that make deep and intimate friendship possible. The stronger those feeling muscles get, the more they can help you through difficult times, as we will see in the next chapter. More than that, strong feeling muscles make it possible to truly appreciate the good times as well.

12

⚬

A Hole in Your Heart: Dealing with Endings and Losses

LEORA HAD JUST TURNED SIXTY. SHE HAD A GOOD job at an animal shelter and was happily married to her third husband, which she said "is the lucky number." Her life with him, as well as with her two children, three grandchildren, and two rescue dogs, was rich and fulfilling. But when one of her best friends died after a long illness, Leora said, "It was almost impossible for me to deal with it. We've been friends forever. Sometimes we didn't see or talk to each other for weeks or even months. But she was always there, always part of my life. She was part of me, and I was part of her. And now that part is gone. It's like I've lost a part of myself."

Grief is a normal reaction to the loss of a friend, but how we grieve varies from person to person. Describing the loss of her close friend and colleague Caroline Knapp, Gail Caldwell writes of the "physical weight of sadness" and adds, "What they never tell you about grief is that missing someone is the easy part."[1] For Caldwell, the feeling of being alone, without Caroline to go through life with her, was like playing a game of catch by herself. "What am I supposed to do here?" she wondered. "My life had made so much sense alongside hers."[2] Without the intimacy they had shared, Caldwell felt as though her own life no longer made sense.

Such a sense of loss can come from less obvious directions as well. Because connections are so important to women, it is not unusual for us to grieve the end of any close friendship, whether it is the result of death, life changes, or an unresolvable dispute. According to the American Psychological Association's Help Center, "Coping with the loss of a close friend or family member may be one of the hardest challenges that many of us face."[3] Like Gail Caldwell, women from all over the world and in different stages of life told me of feeling frightened, lonely, and untethered when a close friend was no longer accessible. These emotions, as Caldwell writes, can have a physical presence in our bodies.

In her memoir *Something More Wonderful: A True Story,* the Australian author Sonia Orchard describes some of the raw feelings that emerged during the year that she and her friend Emma, both only thirty-one years old, dealt with Emma's cancer and impending death. But in many popular treatments, friends' deaths are quickly glossed over. In an episode of the HBO show *Girls,* for instance, after the death of one character, there is a brief discussion between two young women, Jessa and Shoshanna, about whether they have ever experienced the death of a friend. Shoshanna discloses that a friend died in high school, and that she (Shoshanna) was happy because she got to take the girl's place in their friend group. Jessa ignores Shoshanna's revelation and starts to talk unemotionally about the drug overdose of her own friend. Granted, these characters are meant to appear both selfish and superficial, but they also reflect the reality that contemporary media presents tales of death without the accompanying pain we feel in real life.

Yet the feelings, whether we acknowledge them or not, are powerful. Leora put it this way: "I have a very rich life; but I would not be a whole person without my women friends, no matter how many kids, husbands, jobs, or houses I had. My family is important, but my friends are my lifeblood. Losing one of them is like having that blood drain out of me."

The death of a good friend is an obvious loss, but even the death of a woman you have just "been friendly with" can trigger grief. For instance, one woman in her twenties told me about the overwhelming sadness she felt after a friend's sister was killed in a terrorist attack. "Of course it was upsetting," she said, "but I seemed to be overreacting somehow. I was sad about the woman's death, and I felt awful for my friend. And I was horrified about what had happened and that we live in such a violent world. But even though I had liked my friend's sister, I knew that the grief I was feeling wasn't just about my relationship with her. I realized that it was *mortality* that was frightening me. Her death made it clear that life is so fragile — that someone my age, with her whole life ahead of her, can die so suddenly, and in such a violent way." This young woman was responding to the trauma of the attack as much as to the loss of her friend's sister. In her book *Wounded by Reality,* the trauma specialist Ghislaine Boulanger tells us that such catastrophic events can be difficult to process in part because the losses result from people behaving in ways that we do not expect them to behave.[4]

Yet the sudden awareness of our own mortality is a common reaction to the death of a friend, at most any age. Women who lost a friend to illness or an accident when they were young told me, "It was supposed to happen to old people, not to kids our age." A woman in her late fifties echoed many others when she said, "I'm embarrassed that so much of my reaction was self-centered. I lost someone very dear to me, and I couldn't imagine life without her. But I also was suddenly faced with the reality that I would die too. I had known it, of course, but this made it so much more real." And an active eighty-year-old said that the death of her closest friend "reminded me that I have a limited number of years in front of me."

Other Kinds of Loss

Betrayal and rejection, life changes, and chronic illness are only some of the shifts other than death that can take a friend away, sometimes with devastating consequences. As happened with Daphne, who discovered that her husband was having an affair with her best friend, a friend can betray, disappoint, and hurt us so badly that we need to eject the person from our life as protection from further pain.

Losing a friend to death is very different from experiencing the end of a relationship for other reasons. But research tells us that both experiences can have a powerful impact on emotional and physical health.[5] "For six months after my dearest friend died," said one woman, "I had trouble taking care of myself. I didn't want to eat or see anyone. I couldn't take pleasure in anything without her." Many women described some of the same feelings after a friendship ended for other reasons. A saleswoman in a bookstore told me that she felt many of the same emotions after her closest friend ended their relationship in a bitter and hurtful fight "over nothing at all." Afterward she caught "every bug that went through the air. I got the flu twice, more colds than I can remember, and then a case of shingles. I'm normally very healthy. My doctor told me the illnesses were related to stress. The only thing that was stressing me was that my friend was gone."

Such losses often look easier on television. After "best friends forever" Marnie and Hannah have a blowout fight on *Girls,* Marnie quietly fades from the picture for a while. In a later episode, after the two have reunited, with no fanfare and no discussion of what happened, Hannah tells Marnie that she should lower her expectations for their friendship, and Marnie says, "I can't lower them any further." For these two TV friends, hurting each other is part of the equation. In real life, the pain can be too hard to bear.

At times, pain and loss become part of the relationship itself. Hurt and separation are woven through the years of troubled friendship between Elena and Lila in Elena Ferrante's Neapolitan Novels. Even caring acts shared between these two women create pain. Emotional loss binds them to each other. Yet such feelings can also drive a permanent wedge between friends, and despite hostility and conflict, the loss of connection can be overwhelming. This is how it was for Idra, a psychology graduate student, who told me, "My best friend got pregnant by accident, and decided to have the child, even though she and her boyfriend were no longer together. I didn't approve, for lots of reasons. I thought she was throwing her life away. We were still very young, and she could have found another solution for the problem. But I supported her. Her parents were furious with her, kicked her out of the house, and I took her into my tiny studio apartment. I stood by her, gave her money, and even stood up to her parents and tried to get them to see her side of things. They eventually took her back and arranged a marriage for her. I felt like that was also a terrible solution, but it was what she decided to do. I tried to stay friends with her, but I couldn't stomach the choices she made. It didn't happen suddenly, but over time we just didn't have anything to say to each other."

Studies have shown that disappointment in a friend's behavior or feelings that she is "not the person you thought she was" are common reasons that women end friendships.[6] No matter how it looks from the outside, such an ending can be a painful loss for both women. Idra told me, "I heard that her baby was born, but I never saw it. I sent her a baby present, and she sent me a thank-you letter.

So it looks like we're being friendly, but the friendship sort of died. It's odd, though. I still miss her so much."

Friendships also may end when one friend feels that she is giving significantly more and getting significantly less. Women count on mutuality between friends. We sense one another's needs and try to respond appropriately, sometimes subtly and sometimes more directly. And we expect that our close friends will do the same for us. Whether a friend leaves you for unknown reasons or after telling you that she no longer likes you or your lifestyle, you may be left with anger at her, as well as anger at yourself. You may feel that you were not a good enough friend to her, or you may resent her for not giving back to you what you gave to her. The struggle for most of us is to find healthy ways to deal with these conflicting and painful emotions.

"In some ways, it seems to me that it might have been easier if she had died," said a woman who had suffered through a stormy breakup with her best friend. "Of course, I don't wish that had really happened. It would have been horrible. But this way, I'm left with the knowledge that I did something so terrible that she ended things. I feel like I gave everything I had to her, and it wasn't enough. Is that why she ended the friendship? Or did I do something wrong, without knowing it? So she's out there and not forgiving me, and maybe even hating me. And she won't tell me what happened or talk to me at all."

Even if you know why a friend has left, and you know that you have done nothing wrong, that the separation has nothing to do with you, and that your friend still cares about you, her absence from your life can still be difficult. A vivacious empty-nester told me, "I have been part of a very close group of friends since my children were small. We all live in the same community. We have coffee together a couple of times a month, and we talk to each other on the phone every couple of days. We've supported each other through every stage and every sort of problem that can occur in a parent's life, through some of our own drug and alcohol problems, cheating husbands and, at least in one case, a cheating wife; illnesses and death of spouses, parents, and, unfortunately, two children.

"We've also celebrated wonderful events in each other's lives — a success at work, a new job, getting rid of a difficult spouse, finding a new partner, a problem child doing better. There is nothing in my life more comforting than our monthly get-togethers. We meet in one of our homes, order pizza, crack open some beer, kick off our shoes, and talk." Recently, however, one member of the group moved away.

"It makes complete sense," this gregarious woman said. "She's divorced and all alone. Her youngest has moved into his own place with his girlfriend. This community, which is so family-focused, makes her feel sad and lonely. She's ready to meet some single men, and she can't do that here. I don't blame her. I might do the same thing if I was in her place. But I'm so sad. I cannot tell you how much I miss her." Her eyes filled with tears. "We talk on the phone, but it's not the same as being in the same room with her. It feels physical — like she's left a hole in my heart."

There is a reality to the sense that such a loss is physical, even if the feeling is metaphorical. As we have seen, women often speak of feeling "held" by close friends. We provide a sense of safety and security, as well as a feeling of being emotionally solid. Under the best of circumstances, parents provide us with this feeling when we are children. Friends often provide this kind of support as we get older. As the author Molly Castelloe puts it, friends can help us "gather ourselves in a fundamental, emotional way."[7]

This "gathering" is often physical as well as emotional. Women friends nurture us physically, even when we do not literally touch. We express caring, concern, love, and interest with our hands, eyes, face, and voice. We tell our friends that we know how they feel not just with words, but with our physical presence. And because they do the same for us, we feel the loss of that presence when they are no longer with us.

The Stages and Shapes of Grief

In 1969 Elisabeth Kübler-Ross, a Swiss American psychiatrist, introduced the idea that there are five stages that everyone goes through when grieving. Her classic book *On Death and Dying* describes these stages: *denial,* in which we refuse to accept or believe a painful truth; *anger,* which is often misdirected and can include an attempt to blame someone for what may be no one's fault; *bargaining,* or an attempt to make a deal or negotiate a compromise; *depression,* or feelings of hopelessness and helplessness, despair and despondency; and *acceptance,* which involves an awareness that the situation cannot be changed and an effort to adapt in the best possible way, albeit without being unrealistically upbeat. Although researchers and clinicians no longer believe that everyone experiences all of Kübler-Ross's stages, or goes through them in a set order,[8] it can be useful to recognize that grief is complex and that mourning is a process.

Because that process is personal, each of us will mourn the loss of a friend in our own way. Whether you spend extra time with a dying friend or take her child on a special trip, whether you talk about your feelings or avoid the subject of death altogether, will depend on your preferences and your friend's. As with everything else about friendship in women's lives, there is not one right way to mourn.

Most of us move back and forth through the stages of grief. For instance, when Richelle's friend Adeli developed cancer, Richelle organized all of their friends to provide food, transportation, and moral encouragement. Although the cancer was not responding to treatment, Richelle kept telling everyone, "She's tough. She'll kick it. You'll see." Hope is an important part of healing, but it can also be a way of denying reality. Adeli had undergone all of the traditional and alternative treatments that she, her doctors, and her friends had been able to find. Richelle told me, "It was clear that she was not going to live. The doctors said she had about six months. I told myself that they didn't know everything, that people sometimes get better miraculously. I just couldn't accept it. I *wouldn't* accept it." Richelle moved back and forth between denial and bargaining in those early days.

"I don't really believe in God, but I would pray at night and tell Him, 'I'll give her some of the years off of my own life. Take those from me, and give them to her, and I won't complain. Not at all.' Of course, it didn't work." Moving from denial to anger, to acceptance, and then to depression is quite common. Self-criticism and feelings of insecurity are also normal. Richelle told me about her sense that she was not a good enough friend when Adeli was dying. She said, "Everyone told me how amazing I was. I arranged a schedule of visiting and meal preparation with everyone in her circle so that there was always someone at her house and always food for her family. I helped her make a videotape for her daughter, for after Adeli was gone. But still, I can't help feeling like I didn't do enough."

While such guilt may concern something you have legitimately done or not done, it may also be your psyche's effort to convince you that you had more control over a situation than you did. When she unpacked her feelings, Richelle realized that she was "trying to think of some way that I could have stopped Adeli from dying. I don't like it that we don't have any control over death." In a similar way, experiencing depression can be a way of processing angry feelings that you cannot express to your friend; paradoxically, anger directed at an innocent target such as a different friend or a parent, spouse, child — even a pet — may be the psyche's way of avoiding unbearable sadness.

This redirecting of feelings, either inward or outward, is the psyche's way of protecting us from hurt and pain. Yet sometimes this protective mechanism can cause damage to other relationships, to our self-esteem, and to our physical health. The mindfulness expert Elisha Goldstein tells us that it is normal to resist feeling sad, but the effort can leave us tense and irritable. He writes, "Grief is a natural part of the human experience."[9] Allowing ourselves to feel sadness can reduce tension, irritability, and anger. It can also lead to a closer connection to others and a greater ability to take in their compassion. But we can allow the feelings in only when we are ready to do so.

Some losses don't feel like a big deal. We tell ourselves, "That's life," and move on. Others hurt, but before long the injury has healed, and we hardly notice the scar. And then there are losses that feel as if they will never heal. Richelle said that losing Adeli was like losing a part of herself. "I recovered," she said, "but there will always be an empty space where she should be." Loss of a good friend can also destroy the self-confidence and self-assurance we have gained from that person's support — though we may not have realized or acknowledged it before the loss. Numerous women told me of friends they had lost contact with simply because their focus had been elsewhere — on work, children, partners, parents, or a combination of things. College grads and women in their late twenties often spoke of friends who "just have different interests now" because of new jobs, new relationships, and in some cases, new families. One working mom with a new baby said, "But the thing is, even though there are other things filling up my life — important things that I wouldn't give up for the world — I always have this feeling that something's missing. And it's my close girlfriends."

"I can't tell you what exactly is missing," said another woman in her early thirties. "It's almost like reaching out in the night and knowing that my husband is in bed with me. My friends have always just been there." In psychological language, friends often provide us with a secure base, a sense of being grounded enough to live a satisfying, meaningful life.

Another time when many women lose friends is during and after a divorce. "When my husband and I split up," said one woman, echoing the words of many, "I lost a lot of friends. It wasn't so much that they took sides, although some of them did; but a lot of our friends had been his buddies in college first. We were close to the couples, and I thought the women were my friends. But they didn't seem to care enough to carve out a connection with me by myself."

Another woman said, "One of my closest friends started dating again, at the age of forty-seven, and suddenly she was like an adolescent. All she could talk about was the man in her life, how wonderful he was and what a good time they had together. I was glad that she was having a good time. She deserved it after all she went through. But she seemed to stop caring about anything that was going on in my life. I don't think she asked about me for over a year." Another common complaint was that divorced friends who got involved with new boyfriends abandoned the women who had supported them through a difficult phase of life. "It's like I was only important as long as she needed someone to listen to her; but now, she spends all of her time dating, and I don't see or hear from her." The pain of such losses is real. An important connection and a reliable source of support are gone, leaving a sense of personal rejection.

Those who experience divorce may also find that their friendships alter or even disappear. Life changes such as divorce often transform a person's sense of identity, and friends may react by withdrawing. When we no longer feel valued by certain friends, we may wonder whether they ever liked who we truly are. "There's another thing," one recently separated woman added. "I have always felt like I was as important to my friends as they were to me. When I was feeling insecure, I could boost myself up by reminding myself that my friends valued me, even if I didn't always know why. Without them, I've lost that mirror that told me I was a good person."

In NoViolet Bulawayo's novel *We Need New Names,*[10] the narrator leaves her home in Zimbabwe and comes to live in Detroit. She has lost not only a way of life and a group of friends who filled her childhood, but also her identity. She cannot connect with old friends, who feel that she has deserted them and her Zimbabwean roots. At the same time she does not feel a sense of belonging with her new acquaintances. She no longer knows who she is.

The loss of a friend can impact both your feeling of security and your sense of who you are.

What You Can Do

When you lose a friend for any reason, you will likely have some sort of emotional reaction. What the feelings are is less important than how you deal with them. You may feel hurt, guilty, sad, angry, or some combination of these and other feelings. It is important to allow yourself to grieve in your own way. When someone has been a significant part of your life, even a friend you don't see every day, some pain will arise in response to losing that person. Just as a physical wound needs care and gentle attention, so too does an emotional hurt.

Research shows that taking care of yourself physically and maintaining connections with your own support system are important tools in the healing process.[11] For many of us, putting thoughts and feelings into words, whether by expressing them to someone else or by writing them in a journal, can help. These processes get the words out of your head for the moment. Talking about them with someone else can give you the chance to benefit from a perspective different from your own. Writing them down can also give you a different perspective. But research has shown that the act of putting thoughts and feelings into words is beneficial even if you don't change your perspective.[12]

Mindfully attending to yourself is also crucial in these moments. While it is important to unpack your feelings and to accept your own self-criticism when appropriate, remember to be kind. Friendships are a two-way process, and when they go wrong, most often multiple factors are in play. Give yourself room to heal.

The passage of time does promote healing—your grief should eventually become less painful. Many women told me that time and age had also made them realize that there are different kinds of friendships. "The friends I have in my sixties are very different from the ones I had in my twenties," said one woman. "They're not as intense. I don't *have* to talk with them or see them so often. But they're sort of a quiet cushion in the background."

And finally, even when a friend is gone, she is still part of your internal world. In her description of the painful end of a close friendship, the psychologist Jeanne Safer says that she realized she could hold on to the good experiences even while she let go of the connection. She writes, "My lost woman friend is woven into the fabric of my self, where damage and delight intermingle. Now my memories of her are real, three-dimensional—bright as well as dark."[13]

Marilyn Peterson Haus offers yet another way of remembering that a friend is part of you. In her eulogy for her close friend of over forty years, the writer Michelle Gillett, Haus says, "In my last visit with Michelle, I thanked her for being my friend. I told her she would live on in my heart. She said I too would live on with her—and she would remind me of it by rattling things in our house. So now, every time something in our house rattles or creaks, I am reminded that Michelle's warm and generous spirit lives on in me."[14]

This feeling that a friend lives on inside you is called "internalization," which is the psychological term for taking something that is outside you and making it part of yourself. Internalization of qualities of loved ones is one of the ways that we cope with loss. Connecting with that inner space is also part of the joy of friendships between women, the focus of the next chapter.

13

⁓

The Special Joy of "Friendship Wisdom"

L IZ AND EILEEN, SISTERS-IN-LAW WHO HAVE BEEN
friends since middle school, have a special way of communicating. While one talked to me, the other nodded or shook
her head, and shifted her body in response to what her friend was
saying. They made eye contact, shared a smile, or pursed their lips.
"We've been through so much together," said Eileen. "We know one
another inside out." Liz nodded in agreement.

Their friendship epitomized the kind of connection that my colleague Kevin spoke of so longingly at that dinner party, when he
commented that he wished he and his friends could have the deep
emotional bonds that he saw in women's friendships. Yet Liz told

me that she and Eileen seldom talk about "important stuff." Eileen nodded. "Yeah, we're more likely to spend fifteen minutes talking about what we're going to make for dinner and whether or not to let our daughters buy the shoes they are telling us they can't live without."

In fact, many women told me that their conversations with friends were usually about "small things." Could it be that this mutual interest in details is what holds friendships together in difficult times?

The stories of friendship gathered throughout this book come from a wide range of women of different ages, with different backgrounds and different lifestyles, and make it clear that these important connections come in a variety of packages. As I listened to so many women, however, I began to notice a crucial thread that ran quietly through all of the stories: the value that women placed on small, apparently insignificant details. And I found myself wondering if this element, so insignificant that we hardly think to mention it, is in fact the linchpin of these relationships.

A New Definition

Although they did not usually mention it, and perhaps never even thought about it, the women who told me their stories shared a subtle awareness that tiny details are important to their connections to other women. Of course, we women are not alone in sensing this. In Chapter 5 we discussed the American psychoanalyst Harry Stack Sullivan, who believed that psychological understanding and change come from paying attention to the tiny details of everyday life. Based on this belief, Sullivan developed a technique called "detailed inquiry"[1] to help psychotherapists gather key pieces of information about a client's life to help them understand and work more successfully with the individual.

These apparently inconsequential snippets offer major clues to who we are and what makes our lives meaningful. When teens sit and chatter about "nothing" for hours, or old friends break into uncontrollable laughter over a minor incident or look at each other in silent understanding, small elements of experience are quietly drawing us together. Information such as what time the babysitter arrived and what color the new curtains should have been may seem mundane, but the way we communicate them is everything. This "small talk" can convey how we feel: safe or frightened, happy or sad, despondent or hopeful. Details are a vehicle for talking about who we are and what we value.

When women gather in the kitchen for "girl talk" during a dinner party, they are sharing fundamental aspects of life. And when we say, "I know how you feel," whether we are talking about a husband's infidelity, a child's problems, a difficult boss, or a favorite pair of shoes that are pinching a friend's toes, we communicate our understanding that these matters, big and small, are the wellspring of human experience.

A fifty-two-year-old recent widow told me that during her husband's illness and after he died, she found solace with her knitting group, which met once a week at a small shop in her town. "We are all different ages, with different life stories and experiences. We mostly know only each other's first names, and we seldom get together outside of the group. But while we knit, we chat about this and that. I feel soothed by the conversation, even though it's not about anything earth-shattering. Most of them didn't even know what was going on with my husband for a long time. When I did tell them, they were just so comforting and caring. Those hours of talking about unimportant things connected us in a very deep way."

In her memoir *The Bridge Ladies,* Betsy Lerner describes a group of women "of a certain age" who "could play Bridge day in and day out," laughing and talking about nothing at all. She writes, "Conversation cycles through the weather, weekend activities, medical reports, movie reviews, and book reports."[2] Yet though the women never seem to talk about "important things," they understand when a member needs extra support or attention, which they readily supply. For instance, despite the group's unspoken rule against showing off, when one member, Bette, became a grandmother for the first time at the age of eighty, she was "granted special dispensation in the bragging department."[3]

Lily, the eighty-seven-year-old whose friend Marguerite had bossed her around for years, told me, "One of the reasons Marguerite and I stayed friends for so long was that we could talk about anything. We could stay on the phone for hours, and when my husband asked me what we had been talking about, all I could say is 'just this and that.' It was usually just all of the little stuff from our lives. Well, sometimes we would talk about politics, I guess. All I can tell you is that I felt good when we hung up. Relaxed, comfortable, and *full*. I know that sounds strange, but that's the best word I can find for it."

And Melissa, a thirty-one-year-old art teacher, said that she and her best friend, Kim, knew everything there was to know about each other. "We can say anything to each other," she said. Like many women, they could talk for hours about seemingly unimportant things. "We might not talk for a few weeks, and then we'll pick up like we saw each other yesterday," she said. "But we can also talk five days in a row and still find plenty to say. If you listened to us, you'd think we were talking about boring nonsense. But it's part of what keeps us close, I think. We just say whatever random things we're thinking. It's kind of like having a direct line into each other's brains."

An article by Phil Garber, about a group of Muslim and Jewish women who, as part of a national organization, meet monthly in their New Jersey homes, captures this aspect of friendship perfectly: "There is no discussion of the two-state solution, the Gaza Strip, the plight of the Palestinians, or President Donald Trump's plan to relocate the Israeli capital to Jerusalem. Rather, the talk is about the latest trouble with in-laws, whether their children should play football, or how to bake the traditional Jewish bread, challah, or Aish, a traditional Egyptian pocket bread."[4]

The women also study and discuss holy texts of both religions, including the Torah and the Qur'an, but it is the smaller issues that develop trust and connection. One of the organizers of the New Jersey group put it this way: "We sit around a table, share food, and see our points of commonality."

In Times of Trouble

Paying attention to the details may actually help us grow and make important changes. For instance, a young woman told me that she had been stuck in a miserable marriage for several years before she finally went to a therapist for help. The therapist asked if she had talked to any of her friends about the situation. "I was embarrassed," she said. "I didn't want anyone to know what a mess my life was. And I was also afraid I would break down and cry if I did talk about it. Who wants to be around a wet dishrag?" Her therapist encouraged her to pick one friend to talk to about the situation. "She told me that if I cried, it would be okay. My friend would probably figure out a way to deal with it."

The therapist helped her think about which of her acquaintances she could risk sharing with, and they discussed how she would deal with various possible outcomes of opening up. "It was kind of amazing. When I did share what was going on, my friend asked me some really smart questions. She also said that she knew that this was a confusing and kind of overwhelming process, and said she thought I should talk to another woman in our social group, who I only knew slightly, who had gone through something very similar.

"I had been thinking awful things about my husband, but had

been so ashamed of those feelings that I hadn't told anyone, even the therapist, about them. Somehow talking with my friends, who told me some of the stuff they thought about their own husbands and ex-husbands, I was able to say what I'd been thinking about mine. We actually laughed at some of the mean things I had thought were so horrible!

"I didn't suddenly become someone who shares my feelings with everyone. I'll probably never be that kind of person. But those two friends helped me think about the small steps I needed to take to begin the separation process. I think I had been so tied up in my feelings before that I couldn't see what I needed to do, or even what I could do, first."

Women are amazingly practical, and sharing feelings can be part of the process of being practical. The psychoanalyst Robert Stolorow has written that one of the difficulties of traumatic experiences is that we feel alone and isolated. We believe that no one else can understand us. A friend who lets us know that she does understand is also helping us move forward into problem-solving.[5]

Trauma specialists tell us that the capacity to turn to friends in times of trouble helps make us resilient.[6] In her novel *We Need New Names,* NoViolet Bulawayo takes us into the world of a group of children growing up in Zimbabwe; the power of their friendship helps them manage a difficult life in their painfully poor, politically battered community. Then Darling, the narrator, moves to Detroit, Michigan. Although life in America is better for her in terms of physical health and future prospects, the loss of her friends is excruciating. Explaining that she drew on her own experiences for the novel, Bulawayo says, "I am still shadowed by the sacrifices I made to get here. The pain of adjustment not only made me smell my armpits and catch the fine whiff of my outsiderness, but also made me long for my country, even as President Mugabe was bringing Zimbabwe to its knees."

Darling reaches back from the United States to Zimbabwe to

speak via Skype with her friends, but they have changed, and so has she. She makes new friends in Detroit, but they don't know her the way her African friends did. The author says, "Those of us who give up our homelands live with quiet knowledge nestled in our blood like an incurable disease; even as we are here, we are tied to somewhere else."[7]

A new form of therapy for women in areas of Africa and India where no psychotherapists are available is called "the Friendship Bench." Part of the therapy is one-to-one work with a trained non-professional called a "grandmother," who validates a woman's feelings and helps her with realistic problem-solving. But another part of this work involves getting together with others to talk and do craftwork. Bonding over the work is a vehicle for casual conversation, expression of feeling, and a lot of practical advice.

Friendship Wisdom

Research confirms what we know from experience: we change over time, and our friendships change along with us. Studies have also shown that friendship *needs* change over the course of a lifetime.[8] In some cases, as with Liz and Eileen, who first connected in their teens, the friendships evolve as we do. In others, we begin new friendships as old ones dissolve, burst into flames, or slip quietly into the past. In every case, whether you know it or not, you have learned something from your past connections that you bring into your new ones. These different scenarios can take many forms. Women described getting even closer to some friends, winnowing out others, and finding that friends did not have to be deeply attached or perfectly matched to make a meaningful connection.

As Betty Friedan, author of *The Feminine Mystique,* puts it, "Aging is not 'lost youth' but a new stage of opportunity and strength."[9]

An active grandmother told me, "It took me a long time to figure out how to be a good friend. I was shy as a kid, and always felt afraid that other girls didn't like me. I was a smart girl at a time when it wasn't okay to be smart, and I got teased for getting good grades and being 'teacher's pet.' So I mostly kept to myself. Then I went to an all-girls college, which was so competitive that it seemed like all anybody did was study. There was no sense of that 'sisterhood' I've heard so much about at my school. I didn't learn about making friends until I started work after I graduated. An older colleague took me under her wing and became my mentor. I am still close to her, although she has moved out of state. We email and talk on the phone regularly.

"I'll always be grateful to her, not just for what she did for my career, but also for me as a friend. It's maybe surprising that two women of different ages can be friends, but we are. I would say she is probably my closest friend, even though, partly because of her support, I have made other friends over the years. I try to pay what she did for me forward, by mentoring younger women. It's incredibly satisfying to help someone develop. I've become friends with a couple of those women, as well."

Studies show that our friendships not only change as we grow older, but also help us make other life transitions.[10] A recent college grad said that she didn't know what to do when her best friend from college, with whom she had taken an apartment after graduation, told her she was moving in with her boyfriend. "I didn't want to advertise for a new roommate. I didn't want to live with a stranger. But I didn't know anyone else in town." She casually mentioned her problem to a woman at work. "I had categorized her as an acquaintance, not even a 'work friend.' But she asked me how I was doing one day, and I told her the whole sad story. And she stepped right in. She knew someone who was looking for a roommate too, and she said she'd be happy to introduce me. The apartment arrangement didn't work out, but I liked her friend. And I liked her too. Suddenly, I had two friends who were part of my 'grown-up' life. I wasn't a college kid anymore."

We saw this with Daphne, forced to make new friends when her husband and her best friend had an affair. "I have learned from the women in my life now that I'm not just allowed to be vulnerable too, but it's part of true friendship. There's a give and take with these women that I never had with friends when I was younger."

It would seem obvious that such continuity exists for women who remain in contact with friends from childhood, high school, and college. A forty-four-year-old whose mother had died fifteen years earlier told me, "My friends from high school remember my mom. And that helps me stay connected to her."

Yet to get such a sense of continuity, you don't necessarily need to stay friends with your kindergarten classmates. In her book *Kitchen Table Wisdom,* the physician Rachel Naomi Remen speaks of the healing power of storytelling.[11] Talking to new friends about what you have done or how new experiences connect to old ones is a crucial part of developing continuity. In fact, telling your story to a new acquaintance can provide the same kind of link to your own history as does chatting with a childhood buddy. Additionally, as two women share the small details of their personal histories, they connect past experience to the here and now. Relational psychotherapists and evolutionary psychologists agree that telling our story to another person helps us connect to our inner selves in new ways. When done in a way that includes the other person, storytelling can be an opportunity for both people to grow.

When we make new friends at any age, we women tell one another our stories. "Who are you?" we ask, albeit almost always in a subtle and quiet way. "What do you think and feel?" and "How did you get to be the person you are?" An outgoing widow who recently moved to a retirement community to be close to her grown children and grandchildren told me, "I've made a lot of new friends here. I probably never would have gotten to know most of them when I was younger. One in particular has had a rough life. I think her husband hit her, although she doesn't like to talk much about it. It's just from a few things she lets drop here and there that I'm thinking this. We all have almost nothing in common except that we have children who live in this area, which is why we're in this particular place. But we talk to each other about our pasts, and we look out for one another. That's enough to make a good friendship these days."

This woman and many others with whom I spoke shared a "friendship wisdom" that they had developed as they went through the different stages of their lives. While we may treasure old friends, we no longer look for or expect the perfect match and intense mutual understanding of early friendships. We also discover that we have different kinds of friendship needs at different stages of life. Sometimes, to meet these needs, we must make some adjustments to old friendships, and sometimes we must look for new friends. One of the things I heard over and over again, from women all over the world and at many different stages of their lives, was that some relationships had a way of moving from the foreground to the background of their lives, and then back again. If we are lucky, our friendships have a flexibility that allows them to manage these changes. And if we are luckier still, we are also flexible enough to make new friends.

What You Can Do

As we have seen, the joys and the heartbreaks of friendship in women's lives come not from a single kind of relationship, but from the fact that we are wired to connect to others and that we are able to do so in a variety of ways. Something as simple as a shared recipe can connect us to a friend who lives far away or just around the corner. The link resides in the recipe itself, the act of sharing, and the silent companionship of the other woman as we shop for the food, cook it, serve it, and eat it.

The poet and newspaper columnist Michelle Gillett once wrote, "A good friendship is like a good story: enlightening and accessible, familiar and surprising. I want to keep turning the pages. Each time I must put the book down, I look forward to when I can pick it up again."[12] A friend, I would suggest, is someone whose stories interest you, and who is interested in your stories.

Chatting about apparently insignificant life events links us to one another's deepest emotions, in many cases without ever putting the emotions into words. It's a lot easier to do this if you are in the habit of talking from time to time, even about nothing much, than if you haven't spoken in ages. And it's a lot easier to respond to a friend's feelings if you have kept up with the little details of her life. More effort is required if you have to catch up on years of background to understand a current incident in a friend's life.

To me, this is the real truth about the deep connections between women. We pay attention to and connect emotionally over seemingly trivial pieces of information. We provide continuity and stability to one another by being interested in and remembering what may appear to be inconsequential data. As Liz put it, "Eileen and I don't talk to each other every day, and we don't even see each other all that often. We're both busy, and a lot of the time, when we do get together, it's with a big family group, so we can't really visit. But when we haven't had a chance to chat, one of us will call the other. We'll say something like, 'I just wanted to hear your voice.' We can talk for five minutes or an hour, catching up on everything and nothing at all."

If you are looking for a new friend or want to make contact with an old one, don't wait until you have something important to say. Text or email to make a connection, no matter how brief. Even better, call just to chat. You will most likely hear the everyday details of life, some of them interesting, some of them boring. If you share some equally small, insignificant pieces of information about your own life, pat yourself on the back. You are being a friend. This is the wisdom of women's friendships in a nutshell: when we pay attention to the details of one another's lives, everything gets simpler, deeper, and richer.

Acknowledgments

I am deeply grateful to all of the women who shared their stories of friendship with me. Their honesty, courage, and insight are at the heart of this book, and I thank them for that. I have disguised the stories by altering details and changing identifying information in order to protect the privacy of everyone who spoke with me.

I offer thanks, of course, to my wonderful friends, who enrich my life and whose essence is on every page of this book. Their support and their enthusiasm for this project were boundless and inspirational.

Many thanks also to my terrific agent and friend Judith Riven, who has supported and inspired me since she received the first draft of my first book; Deanne Urmy, my amazing, perceptive, insightful, and incredibly hardworking editor at Houghton Mifflin Harcourt; Jenny Xu, a talented and extremely helpful editorial assistant at HMH; Susanna Brougham, who brought her knowledge and impeccable attention to detail to the project; Susan Schwartz, copyeditor par excellence; Betty Kramer, whose expert eye always sees a little something extra; Nicola von Schreiber, who provided support and artistic guidance; Cynthia Medalie, who offered advice, guidance, and hand-holding; and Miriam Ross, who directed me to important material on women's issues.

Numerous people recommended books, films, television shows, websites and web series, art exhibits, plays, and areas of research that broadened and deepened my thinking about women's friendships, and I thank them all!

I also cannot express enough thanks to the wonderful staff at Mason Library in Great Barrington, Massachusetts, who provided incredible assistance with research and who never complained, no matter how difficult my request.

This is a book about women, but it would never have been written without the help of some men, in particular Dr. David Barth, Dr. Rick Barth, and Simon Warren. Crucial support also came from the incredible women in my family: Denise Barth, Abbey Barth, Betty Gai, Blair Warren, Nancy Dixon, Cynthia Coleman, Dr. Joan Warren, Nancy Davis, Courtney Dixon, and Rhoda Jacoby. My heartfelt thanks to all of them.

And of course, many, many thanks to my beloved husband, Joel. Without your love, patience, and encouragement, none of this would have been possible.

Notes

INTRODUCTION

1. Luise Eichenbaum and Susie Orbach are feminists, psychotherapists, and authors who founded the Women's Therapy Center in New York City.

1. HOW SHOULD A FRIENDSHIP BEGIN?

1. C. Wrzus, M. Hänel, J. Wagner, and F. Neyer, "Social Network Changes and Life Events Across the Life Span: A Meta-Analysis," *Psychological Bulletin* 139 (2013): 53–80, doi:10.1037/a0028601.
2. A. Williams, "Friends of a Certain Age: Why Is It Hard to Make Friends over 30?" *New York Times* (July 13, 2012).
3. G. Mollenhorst, B. Völker, and H. Flap, "Changes in Personal Relationships: How Social Contexts Affect the Emergence and Discontinuation of Relationships," *Social Networks* 37 (May 2014): 65–80.
4. Elena Ferrante, *Those Who Leave and Those Who Stay* (New York: Europa Editions, 2014).
5. Pat O'Connor, "Women's Friendships in a Post-Modern World," *Placing Friendship in Context,* R. Adams and G. Allan (Eds.) (London: Cambridge University Press, 1999), 117–135; Mollenhorst, Völker, and Flap, "Changes in Personal Relationships."
6. Some other popular shows offering more nuanced images of women's friendships: *Bridesmaids, UnReal,* and *Gilmore Girls.*
7. C. S. Lewis, *The Voyage of the Dawn Treader* (New York: Harper Collins, 2008 edition), 233.
8. H. Kohut, *The Analysis of the Self: A Systematic Approach to the Psychoanalytic*

Treatment of Narcissistic Personality Disorders (Chicago: University Of Chicago Press, 2009).

9. J. Bowlby, *A Secure Base: Parent-Child Attachment and Healthy Human Development* (New York: Basic Books, 1988).

10. Harville Hendrix, *Getting the Love You Want: A Guide for Couples* (New York: St. Martin's Griffin Press, 2005).

11. Mollenhorst, Völker, and Flap, "Changes in Personal Relationships."

12. Howard Bacal, *Optimal Responsiveness: How Therapists Heal Their Patients* (Lanham, MD: Jason Aronson, 1998).

13. Brené Brown, *Daring Greatly: How the Courage to Be Vulnerable Transforms the Way We Live, Love, Parent, and Lead* (New York: Penguin Group, 2012).

14. S. T. Charles and L. L. Carstensen, "Social and Emotional Aging," *Annual Review of Psychology* 61 (2010), www.annualreviews.org; O' Connor, "Women's Friendships in a Post-Modern World"; Mollenhorst, Völker, and Flap, "Changes in Personal Relationships."

15. https://www.buzzfeed.com/chelseypippin/17-apps-that-can-actually-improve-your-social-life?utm_term=.whEa93jyk#.pq2QqgX8w.

2. WHAT ARE WOMEN'S FRIENDSHIPS?

1. Sandy Sheehy, *Connecting: The Enduring Power of Female Friendship* (New York: HarperCollins, 2000), 30–31.

2. Geoffrey Greif, "Men's and Women's Friendships: Do Men and Women Differ in How They Define Friendships?" PsychologyToday.com (2008), https://www.psychologytoday.com/blog/buddy-system/200811/mens-and-womens-friendships.

3. "61% of Adult Women Agree Having Close Friendships Improves Health," http://www.prnewswire.com/news-releases/61-of-adult-women-agree-having-close-friendships-improves-health-54998887.html.

4. Pat O'Connor, *Friendships Between Women: A Critical Review* (New York: The Guilford Press, 1992).

5. Ibid.; Social Issues Research Centre, "Girl Talk: The New Rules of Female Friendship and Communication," Oxford, UK, n.d. Research commissioned by Diet Coke.

6. Alexander Nehamas, *On Friendship* (New York: Basic Books, 2016), 4.

7. Allison Amend, *Enchanted Islands* (New York: Random House, 2016), 13.

8. Daniel Goleman, "Are Women More Emotionally Intelligent than Men?" *Psychology Today* (2011), https://www.psychologytoday.com/blog/the-brain-and-emotional-intelligence/201104/are-women-more-emotionally-intelligent-men; Jude Cassidy and Phillip R. Shaver, eds., *Handbook of Attachment: Theory, Research, and Clinical Applications,* 2nd ed. (New York: Guilford Press, 2010).

9. Goleman, "Are Women More Emotionally Intelligent than Men?"

10. Emiliana R. Simon-Thomas, "Are Women More Empathic than Men?" *Greater Good,* June 1, 2007.

11. Deborah Tannen, *You Just Don't Understand: Women and Men in Conversation* (New York: William Morrow, 2007).

12. O'Connor, "Women's Friendships in a Post-Modern World"; Peter Marsh, Simon Bradley, Carol Love, Patrick Alexander, and Roger Norham, *Belonging* (Oxford, UK: Social Issues Research Centre, July 2007. Research commissioned by the Automobile Association).

13. Louis Sander, "Identity and the Experience of Specificity in a Process of Recognition: Commentary on Seligman and Shanok," *Psychoanalytic Dialogues,* 5 (1995): 579–593.

14. D. W. Winnicott, *Through Paediatrics to Psycho-Analysis,* (London: Hogarth Press and the Institute of Psycho-Analysis, 1975).

15. Jack van Honk, Dennis J. Schutter, Peter A. Bos, Anne-Wil Kruijt, Eef G. Lentjes, and Simon Baron-Cohen, "Testosterone Administration Impairs Cognitive Empathy in Women Depending on Second-to-Fourth Digit Ratio," *Proceedings of the National Academy of Science* 108, no. 8 (February 22, 2011). https://www.researchgate.net/profile/Peter_Bos/publication/49817064_Testosterone_administration_impairs_cognitive_empathy_in_women_depending_on_second-to-fourth_digit_ratio/links/0912f50b5d773ca9e0000000.pdf.

16. Kelly Campbell, Nicole Holderness, and Matt Riggs, "Friendship Chemistry: An Examination of Underlying Factors," *Social Science Journal* 52 (2015): 239–247, http://dx.doi.org/10.1016/j.soscij.2015.01.005.

17. Stephen Mitchell, *Relational Concepts in Psychoanalysis: An Integration* (Boston: Harvard University Press, 1988).

18. O' Connor, "Women's Friendships in a Post-Modern World."

19. Jeffrey Zaslow, *The Girls from Ames* (New York: Gotham Books, 2009), 270.

20. Krystal D'Costa, "Catfishing: The Truth About Deception Online," *Scientific American* (2014), http://blogs.scientificamerican.com/anthropology-in-practice/catfishing-the-truth-about-deception-online/.

21. National Public Radio, "Teen Girls Flip the Negative Script on Social Media" (2016), http://www.npr.org/sections/alltechconsidered/2016/03/24/470686073/teengirls-flip-the-negative-script-on-social-media (accessed March 24, 2016).

22. Nancy Jo Sales, *American Girls: Social Media and the Secret Lives of Teenagers* (New York: Vintage Publishers, 2016); danah boyd, *It's Complicated: The Social Lives of Networked Teens* (New Haven, CT: Yale University Press, 2014); D.L.G. Borzekowski, S. Schenk, J. L. Wilson, and R. Peebles, "e-Ana and e-Mia: A Content Analysis of Pro-ED Websites," *American Journal of Public Health* 100 (2010): 1526–1534.

23. Sara Coughlin, "Your Facebook Friends' Finances Might Matter More Than You Think," *Refinery29* (August 5, 2015), http://www.refinery29.com/2015/08/91879/facebook-friends-credit-rating.

24. This is such a common story that a television cable company has developed an advertisement around it. Two men work on a cable-related problem. When they are done, they clearly have nothing to talk about. Their wives, however, have been chatting the whole time and are still chatting while the men look at each other in silence. Gesturing to the women, one of the men says to the other, "So, are they ready to wrap things up here?"

3. FRIENDS AND FAMILY:
ONE WE CHOOSE, ONE WE DON'T

1. Jay McInerney, *The Last of the Savages* (New York: Vintage Books, 1997), 3.

2. Matthew D. Lieberman, *Social: Why Our Brains Are Wired to Connect* (New York: Random House, 2013), 293.

3. Zaslow, *The Girls from Ames.*

4. Erik H. Erikson, *Identity and the Life Cycle* (New York: International Universities Press, 1959).

5. Allan Schore, *Affect Regulation and the Origin of the Self: The Neurobiology of Emotional Development* (Oxford, UK: Taylor and Francis/Routledge, 2016).

6. Natalie Madorsky Elman and Eileen Kennedy-Moore, *The Unwritten Rules of Friendship: Simple Strategies to Help Your Child Make Friends* (New York: Little, Brown, 2003).

7. Tiffany Field, "Attachment and Separation in Young Children," *Annual Review of Psychology* 47 (1996), 541–561.

8. Susan T. Charles and Laura L. Carstensen, "Social and Emotional Aging," *Annual Review of Psychology* 61 (2009): 383–409.

9. J. Weiss and H. Sampson, *The Psychoanalytic Process: Theory, Clinical Observation, and Empirical Research* (New York: Guilford Press, 1986).

10. Mark L. Laudenslager, Teresa L. Simoneau, Sam Philips, Patrick Benitez, Crystal Natvig, and Steve Cole, "A Randomized Controlled Pilot Study of Inflammatory Gene Expression in Response to a Stress Management Intervention for Stem Cell Transplant Caregivers," *Journal of Behavioral Medicine* 39 (2016): 346–354.

11. R. B. Williams, J. C. Barefoot, R. M. Califf, T. L. Haney, W. B. Saunders, D. B. Pryor, M. A. Hlatky, I. C. Siegler, and D. B. Mark, "Prognostic Importance of Social and Economic Resources Among Medically Treated Patients with Angiographically Documented Coronary Artery Disease," *Journal of the American Medical Association* 267 (1992): 520–524.

12. C. H. Kroenke, Y. L. Michael, X. O. Shu, E. M. Poole, M. L. Kwan, S. Nechuta, B. J. Caan, J. P. Pierce, and W. Y. Chen, "Post-Diagnosis Social Networks, and Lifestyle and Treatment Factors in the After Breast Cancer Pooling Project," *Psychooncology* (January 8, 2016), doi:10.1002/pon.4059.

13. S. E. Taylor, L. C. Klein, B. P. Lewis, T. L. Gruenewald, R.A.R. Gurung, and J. A. Updegraff, "Behavioral Responses to Stress in Females: Tend-and-Befriend, Not Fight-or-Flight," *Psychological Review* 107 (2000): 411–429.

14. Steven Reinberg, "Loneliness May Sabotage Breast Cancer Survival, Study Finds," *HealthDay,* December 12, 2016. http://www.cbsnews.com/news/loneliness-may-sabotage-breast-cancer-survival-study-finds/.

15. Daniel J. Siegel, *The Developing Mind: How Relationships and the Brain Interact to Shape Who We Are,* 2nd ed. (New York: Guilford Press, 2015); Daniel Goleman, *Emotional Intelligence: Why It Can Matter More Than IQ,* 10th anniversary ed. (New York: Bantam Books, 2005).

16. Rivka Galchen, "My Friends' Moms," *The New Yorker* (May 7, 2016), http://www.newyorker.com/books/page-turner/my-friends-moms.

17. Daniel Goleman, *Emotional Intelligence: Why It Can Matter More Than IQ.*

4. DISILLUSIONMENT, BETRAYAL, AND REJECTION

1. Jan Yager, *When Friendship Hurts: How to Deal with Friends Who Betray, Abandon, or Wound You* (New York: Touchstone Books, 2010).

2. https://www.ahdictionary.com/word/search.html?q=betray&submit.x=52&submit.y=24.

3. Warren H. Jones, Danny S. Moore, Arianne Schratter, and Laura A. Negel, "Interpersonal Transgressions and Betrayals," *Behaving Badly: Aversive Behaviors in Interpersonal Relationships,* Robin M. Kowalski (Ed.) (Washington, D.C.: American Psychological Association, 2001): 233–256; Julie Fitness, "Betrayal, Rejection, Revenge, and Forgiveness: An Interpersonal Script Approach," *Interpersonal Rejection,* M. Leary (Ed.) (New York: Oxford University Press, 2001), 73–103; Mark R. Leary, Carrie Springer, Laura Negel, Emily Ansell, and Kelly Evans, "The Causes, Phenomenology, and Consequences of Hurt Feelings," *Journal of Personality and Social Psychology* 74 (1998): 1225–1237, http://dx.doi.org/10.1037/0022-3514.74.5.1225.

4. Fitness, "Betrayal, Rejection, Revenge, and Forgiveness."

5. Jenny De Jong Gierveld, Pearl A. Dykstra, and Niels Schenk, "Living Arrangements, Intergenerational Support Types, and Older Adult Loneliness in Eastern and Western Europe," *Demographic Research* 27 (2012), doi:10.4054/DemRes.2012.27.7.

6. *Orange Is the New Black,* season 4, episode 8, 2014.

7. Elena Ferrante, *The Story of a New Name: Neapolitan Novels, Book Two* (New York: Penguin, 2013), 6.

8. Jane Austen, *Northanger Abbey* (New York: Penguin Classics, 2003), chapter 6. You can also watch Carey Mulligan as she says these words in the 2007 film version.

9. Robert Stolorow, *Trauma and Human Existence* (New York: Routledge, 2007).

10. Luise Eichenbaum and Susie Orbach, *Between Women: Love, Envy, and Competition in Women's Friendships* (New York: Penguin Books, 1989).

11. Harriet Lerner, *The Dance of Connection: How to Talk to Someone When You're Mad, Hurt, Frustrated, Insulted, Betrayed, or Desperate* (New York: William Morrow, 2002).

12. E. Georges, "A Cultural and Historical Perspective on Confession," *Emotion, Disclosure, and Health,* J. W. Pennebaker (Ed.) (Washington, D.C.: American Psychological Association, 1995): 11–22.

13. Jeanne Safer, *Forgiving and Not Forgiving: Why Sometimes It's Better Not to Forgive* (New York: HarperCollins, 2010); Lerner, *The Dance of Connection.*

14. Roy F. Baumeister, *Evil: Inside Human Violence and Cruelty* (New York: W. H. Freeman Publishers, 1996); Robert Bies and Thomas Tripp, "Beyond Distrust: 'Getting Even' and the Need for Revenge," *Trust in Organizations: Frontiers in Theory and Research,* R. M. Kramer and T. R. Tyler (Eds.) (Thousand Oaks, CA: Sage Publications, 1996): 246–260.

15. Frederic Luskin, *Forgive for Good: A Proven Prescription for Health and Happiness* (New York: HarperOne, 2001).

5. THE JOY OF BELONGING, THE PAIN OF EXCLUSION: GROUPS, CLUBS, AND CLIQUES

1. D. R. Forsyth, *Group Dynamics,* 6th ed. (Belmont, CA: Wadsworth Cengage Learning, 2014).

2. I. Fishman, R. Ng, and U. Bellugi, "Do Extraverts Process Social Stimuli Differently from Introverts? *Cognitive Neuroscience* 2, (2011): 67–73, http://doi.org/10.1080/17588928.2010.527434.

3. Susan T. Fiske, *Social Beings: Core Motives in Social Psychology* (Hoboken, NJ: John Wiley and Sons, 2010).

4. Ibid.

5. R. M. Kertzner, I. H. Meyer, D. M. Frost, and M. J. Stirratt, "Social and Psychological Well-Being in Lesbians, Gay Men, and Bisexuals: The Effects of Race, Gender, Age, and Sexual Identity," *American Journal of Orthopsychiatry* 79 (2009): 500–510; B. J. Gillespie, D. Frederick, L. Harari, and C. Grov, "Homophily, Close Friendship, and Life Satisfaction Among Gay, Lesbian, Heterosexual, and Bisexual Men and Women," *PLoS ONE* 10 (2015), http://doi.org/10.1371/journal.pone.0128900.

6. From an interview on NPR's *Weekend Edition:* http://www.npr.org/2016/07/10/485432457/reflecting-on-recent-fatal-police-shootings-

children-s-author-kwame-alexander-fo; see also some of his books at http://www.amazon.com/Kwame-Alexander/e/B001K8ZOJ8.

7. Naomi Novik, *Uprooted* (New York: Del Rey Publishers, 2016).
8. Melanie Suchet, "Face to Face," *Psychoanalytic Dialogues* 20 (2010): 158–171.
9. Heinz Kohut, *The Analysis of the Self* (Chicago: University of Chicago Press, 1971/2009).
10. Erikson, *Identity and the Life Cycle*.
11. Carlin Flora, "The Mixed Bag Buddy [And Other Friendship Conundrums]," *Psychology Today* (January 2, 2013), https://www.psychologyto day.com/articles/201301/the-mixed-bag-buddy-and-other-friendship-conundrums?collection=1087184.
12. Novick, *Uprooted,* 420.

6. HOW MANY FRIENDS DO YOU NEED?

1. Alex Morritt, *Impromptu Scribe* (Paxanax Press, 2014).
2. D. Umberson and J. K. Montez, "Social Relationships and Health: A Flashpoint for Health Policy," *Journal of Health and Social Behavior* 51 (2010), http://doi.org/10.1177/0022146510383501; J. S. House, K. R. Landis, and D. Umberson, "Social Relationships and Health," *Science* 29 (July 1988): 540–545.
3. Schore, *Affect Regulation and the Origin of the Self;* Charles and Carstensen, "Social and Emotional Aging"; Umberson and Montez, "Social Relationships and Health"; House, Landis, and Umberson, "Social Relationships and Health."
4. Debra Umberson, Robert Crosnoe, and Corinne Reczek, "Social Relationships and Health Behaviors Across the Life Course," *Annual Review of Sociology* 36 (2010): 139–157.
5. Janet Flanner, "Dearest Edith," Profiles, *The New Yorker* (March 2, 1929), http://www.newyorker.com/magazine/1929/03/02/dearest-edith.
6. Susan Cain, *Quiet: The Power of Introverts in a World That Can't Stop Talking* (New York: Broadway Books, 2013), 11. Cain tells us that introverts who changed the world include Eleanor Roosevelt, Rosa Parks, Chopin, Gandhi, Dr. Seuss, Steve Wozniak, Al Gore, and Warren Buffett.
7. H. H. Fung, L. L. Carstensen, and F. R. Lang. "Age-Related Patterns in Social Networks Among European Americans and African Americans: Implications for Socioemotional Selectivity Across the Life Span," *International Journal of Aging and Human Development* 52 (2001): 185–206; H. H. Fung, F. S. Stoeber, D. Y. Yeung, and F. R. Lang, "Cultural Specificity of Socioemotional Selectivity: Age Differences in Social Network Composition Among Germans and Hong Kong Chinese," *Journal of Gerontology Series B: Psychological Sciences and Social Sciences* 63B (2008): 156–164.

8. Stephanie Pappas, "7 Ways Friendships Are Great for Your Health," *Live Science* (January 8, 2016), http://www.livescience.com/53315-how-friend-ships-are-good-for-your-health.html.

9. Jenna Wortham, "Feel Like a Wallflower? Maybe It's Your Facebook Wall," *New York Times* (April 10, 2011), http://www.nytimes.com/2011/04/10/business/10ping.html.

10. Rosie Boycott, "Can't Pick a Dress or a Holiday in Case a Friend Does Better? You've Got a Modern Malaise Called FOMO (Fear Of Missing Out)," *The Daily Mail* (April 29, 2011), http://www.dailymail.co.uk/femail/article-1381788/Have-got-modern-malaise-called-FOMO-Fear-Of-Missing-Out.html#ixzz4Qe3vNMmP.

11. Eichenbaum and Orbach, *Between Women,* 172.

12. Cheryl L. Carmichael, Harry T. Reis, and Paul R. Duberstein, "In Your 20s It's Quantity, in Your 30s It's Quality: The Prognostic Value of Social Activity Across 30 Years of Adulthood," *Psychology and Aging* 30, (2015): 95–105.

13. Paula Hawkins, "100 Women 2016: Are Difficult Friendships Better?" *BBC News Magazine* (November 21, 2016), http://www.bbc.com/news/magazine-37769662.

14. Mollenhorst, Völker, and Flap, "Changes in Personal Relationships."

15. Hawkins, "Are Difficult Friendships Better?"

16. Peter Fonagy, *Attachment Theory and Psychoanalysis* (New York: Penguin Random House, 2010).

17. Heinz Kohut, *The Analysis of the Self.*

18. Jessica Benjamin, *The Bonds of Love* (New York: Pantheon Books, 1988).

19. Stolorow, *Trauma and Human Existence.*

20. Lieberman, *Social;* Pappas, "7 Ways Friendships Are Great for Your Health"; Robert Putnam, *Bowling Alone: The Collapse and Revival of American Community* (New York: Touchstone Books, 2001).

7. SHOULD FRIENDS GIVE ADVICE TO FRIENDS?

1. Julie Bort, "The 10 Most Controversial Things Sheryl Sandberg Just Said About Women," *Business Insider* (March 10, 2013), http://www.businessinsider.com/sandberg-controversial-quotes-2013-3.

2. Suzanne Lucas, "Bossiness Is Not a Leadership Trait, No Matter What Sheryl Sandberg Says," February 13, 2014, http://www.inc.com/suzanne-lucas/bossiness-is-not-a-leadership-trait-no-matter-what-sheryl-sandberg-says.html.

3. Edith Wharton, *The Custom of the Country* (New York: Vintage Publishers, 2012), 136.

4. http://exceptionmag.com/19551/6-compelling-reasons-taylor-swift-is-effectively-squadgoals/.

5. Lindsay Putnam, "Taylor Swift 'Squad' Has Become a Cult," *New York Post,* September 1, 2015, http://nypost.com/2015/09/01/taylor-swifts-squad-has-become-a-cult/.

6. Amy Zimmerman, "Is America Turning on Taylor Swift?," *Daily Beast,* August 12, 2015, http://www.thedailybeast.com/articles/2015/08/12/is-america-turning-on-taylor-swift.html.

7. Catherine Kast, "Naomi Campbell on Her Supermodel Crew: 'We Were Never a Squad, We Were Just Friends,'" *People,* April 8, 2016, http://people.com/style/naomi-campbell-on-her-supermodel-crew-we-were-never-a-squad-we-were-just-friends/.

8. Liane Moriarty, *Big Little Lies* (New York: Berkeley Publishers, 2014), 342.

9. Gabrielle Levy, "Hillary Clinton Lets Humans of New York See Her Softer Side," *US News* (September 9, 2016), http://www.usnews.com/news/articles/2016-09-09/hillary-clinton-lets-humans-of-new-york-see-her-softer-side.

10. Susan Albers, "Powerful Tool to Stop Emotional Eating," PsychologyToday.com (December 15, 2015), https://www.psychologytoday.com/blog/comfort-cravings/201512/powerful-tool-stop-emotional-eating; Liz Pryor, "Life Tips from Advice Guru Liz Pryor: Standing Up to Bossy Behavior," ABC News (June 28, 2011), http://abcnews.go.com/GMA/life-tips-advice-guru-liz-pryor-standing-bossy/story?id=13947104; Diane Barth, "What's the Best Way to Handle a Know-It-All?" PsychologyToday.com (December 21, 2013), https://www.psychologytoday.com/blog/the-couch/201312/what-s-the-best-way-handle-know-it-all.

11. Meg Selig, "9 Ways to Be There for a Friend, Without Giving Advice," PsychologyToday.com (October 24, 2014), https://www.psychologytoday.com/blog/changepower/201410/9-ways-be-there-friend-without-giving-advice.

12. Thomas G. Plante, "Giving People Advice Rarely Helps. This Does," *Psychology Today* (July 15, 2014), https://www.psychologytoday.com/blog/do-the-right-thing/201407/giving-people-advice-rarely-works-does.

8. WITH FRIENDS LIKE THIS, WHO NEEDS ENEMIES? COMPETITION BETWEEN FRIENDS

1. Research has indicated that there may be a biological-genetic link between alcoholism and some types of eating disorders. Amy Baker Dennis and Bethany Helfman, "Substance Abuse and Eating Disorders: What Parents and Families Need to Know," *NEDA* (2012) https://www.nationaleatingdisorders.org/substance-abuse-and-eating-disorders; Adrienne Ressler, "Insatiable Hungers: Eating Disorders and Substance Abuse," *Social Work Today* 8 (2008): 30.

This is a subject I have studied for years. Here are two of my articles:

F. D. Barth, "Alexithymia, Affect Regulation, and Binge Drinking in College Students," *Journal of College Student Psychotherapy* 29 (2015): 132–146; "Listening to Words, Hearing Feelings: Links Between Eating Disorders and Alexithymia," *Clinical Social Work Journal Online* (2015).

2. Adrienne Harris, "Aggression: Pleasures and Dangers," *Psychoanalytic Inquiry* 18 (1998): 31–44.
3. Ruth Moulton, "Professional Success: A Conflict for Women," *Psychoanalysis and Women: Contemporary Reappraisals,* J. Alpert (Ed.) (Hillsdale, NJ, and London: Analytic Press, 1986), 161–182.
4. Deborah Tannen, *You're the Only One I Can Tell: Inside the Language of Women's Friendships* (New York: Ballantine Books, 2017), 105.
5. Sheryl Sandberg, *Lean In: Women, Work, and the Will to Lead* (New York: Knopf, 2013).
6. Eichenbaum and Orbach, *Between Women.*
7. Rebecca Johnson, "Why Serena Williams Is Best Friends with Her Fiercest Competitor," Vogue.com (March 21, 2015), http://www.vogue.com/12135713/serena-williams-april-cover-caroline-wozniacki/.
8. Anita Diamant, *The Red Tent* (New York: St. Martin's Press, 2010).
9. Adam Phillips, *One Way and Another: New and Selected Essays* (London: Hamish Hamilton Ltd., 2013).
10. Rachel Anne Binns Terrill, "Inside NFL Marriages: A Seven-Year Ethnographic Study of Love and Marriage in Professional Football" (University of South Florida: Scholar Commons, Graduate Theses and Dissertations, January 2012), 100, luvrofwrds@aol.com.
11. Moriarty, *Big Little Lies,* 52–53.
12. Melanie Klein, *Envy and Gratitude and Other Works, 1946–1963* (New York: Simon and Schuster, 1975).
13. Yager, *When Friendship Hurts.*
14. Virginia Demos, "Basic Human Priorities Reconsidered," *Annals of Psychoanalysis* 36 (2008): 246–265.
15. Grace Reader, "Coach Pat Summitt's 10 Most Inspirational Quotes," Entrepreneur.com (June 28, 2016), https://www.entrepreneur.com/article/278277.
16. Luise Eichenbaum and Susie Orbach, *Understanding Women: A Feminist Psychoanalytic Approach* (Seattle: Amazon Digital Services, 2013), 190.
17. Mary McCarthy, *The Group* (Boston and New York: Mariner Books, 1991 edition), 276.

9. SEXUAL TENSION IN WOMEN'S FRIENDSHIPS

1. E. Wilkinson, "Love in the Multitude?: A Feminist Critique of Love as a Political Concept," *Love: A Question for Feminism in the Twenty-first Cen-*

tury, A. G. Jónasdóttir and A. Ferguson (Eds.) (New York: Routledge, 2014), 237–249.

2. *Sex and the City,* episode 51, "Defining Moments."

3. Trish Bendix, "Madonna's Most Lesbian Moments," *After Ellen,* August 16, 2013, http://www.afterellen.com/people/194564-madonnas-most-lesbian -moments; Kathy Beige, "Christina Aguilar: Girls Are Nice to Kiss," *Lesbian Life,* n.d., http://lesbianlife.about.com/cs/famouslesbians/p/Christina.htm.

4. G. Rieger, R. C. Savin-Williams, M. L. Chivers, and J. M. Bailey, "Sexual Arousal and Masculinity-Femininity of Women," *Journal of Personality and Social Psychology* 111, (2016): 265–283, doi:10.1037/pspp0000077.

5. Shere Hite, *The Hite Report: A National Study of Female Sexuality* (London: Macmillan, 1976).

6. Suzanna M. Rose and Michelle M. Hospital, "Women's Love and Friendship," *APA Handbook of the Psychology of Women,* Cheryl B. Travis and Jacquelyn W. White (Eds.) (Washington, DC: American Psychological Association, 2017).

7. Melanie Canterberry and Omri Gillath, "Attachment and Caregiving," *The Wiley-Blackwell Handbook of Couples and Family Relationships,* Patricia Noller and Gery C. Karantzas (Eds.) (Malden, MA, and Oxford, UK: Wiley-Blackwell, 2012).

8. A. Chandra, W. D. Mosher, C. Copen, and C. Sionean, "Sexual Behavior, Sexual Attraction, and Sexual Identity in the United States: Data from the 2006–2008 National Survey of Family Growth," *National Health Statistics Reports* 36 (2011); Suzanne Zalewski, "Getting Messed Up to Hook Up: The Role of Alcohol in College Students' 'Casual' Sexual Encounters," PsychologyToday. com (2011), https://www.psychologytoday.com/blog/partying-101/201106/ getting-messed-hook-the-role-alcohol-in-college-students-casual-sexual; Kathleen A. Bogle, *Hooking Up: Sex, Dating, and Relationships on Campus* (New York: New York University Press, 2008).

9. Jean M. Twenge, Ryne A. Sherman, and Brooke E. Wells, "Sexual Inactivity During Young Adulthood Is More Common Among U.S. Millennials and iGen: Age, Period, and Cohort Effects on Having No Sexual Partners After Age 18," *Archives of Sexual Behavior* (2016), doi:10.1007/s10508-016-0798-z.

10. Emma Straub, *Modern Lovers* (New York: Riverhead Books, 2016).

11. K. B. Davis, *Factors in the Sex Life of Twenty-two Hundred Women* (New York: Arno Press and the *New York Times,* 1972; original work published 1929).

12. A. L. Bleske and D. M. Buss, "Can Men and Women Be Just Friends? *Personal Relationships* 7 (2000): 131–151; April Bleske-Rechek et al., "Benefit or Burden? Attraction in Cross-Sex Friendship," *Journal of Social and Personal Relationships* 29 (2012): 569, doi:10.1177/0265407512443611, http://isites.harvard.edu/fs/docs/icb.topic1214378.files/February%2025%20Readings/ Bleske-Rechek%20et%20al%202012.pdf

13. Justin J. Lehmiller, Laura E. VanderDrift, and Janice R. Kelly, "Sex Differences in Approaching Friends with Benefits Relationships." *Journal of Sex Research* 48 (2011).

14. S. W. Duck and P. H. Wright, "Re-examining Gender Differences in Same-Gender Friendships," *Sex Roles* 28 (1993): 1–19; L. A. Sapadin, "Friendship and Gender: Perspectives of Professional Men and Women," *Journal of Social and Personal Relationships* 6 (1988): 387–403.

15. Bleske and Buss, "Can Men and Women Be Just Friends?"

16. John F. Helliwell and Shawn Grover, "How's Life At Home?," National Bureau of Economic Research working paper, December 14, http://www.nber.org/papers/w20794.

17. http://www.huffingtonpost.com/2015/01/09-married-people-happier-_n_6436420.html.

18. Fern L. Johnson, "Friendships Among Women: Closeness in Dialogue," *Gendered Relationships,* Julia T. Wood (Ed.) (Houston, TX: Mayfield Publisher, 1996).

19. Julia T. Wood, *Gendered Lives: Communication, Gender, and Culture* (Belmont, CA: Wadsworth Publishers, 1994).

20. Michelle Huston and Pepper Schwartz, "Gendered Dynamics in the Romantic Relationships of Lesbians and Gay Men," *Gendered Relationships,* Julia T. Wood (Ed.) (Houston, TX: Mayfield Publisher, 1996).

21. Lieberman, *Social.*

22. Allan Schore, *Affect Regulation and the Origin of the Self: The Neurobiology of Emotional Development;* Daniel Siegel, *The Developing Mind: How Relationships and the Brain Interact to Shape Who We Are.*

23. Tannen, *You're the Only One I Can Tell.*

24. Nicholas Christakis and James Fowler, *Connected: The Surprising Power of Our Social Networks and How They Shape Our Lives* (New York: Little, Brown and Company, 2009).

10. DO GOOD BOUNDARIES MAKE BAD FRIENDS?

1. O'Connor, *Friendships Between Women.*

2. https://www.ahdictionary.com/word/search.html?q=boundary&submit.x=30&submit.y=26.

3. https://www.ahdictionary.com/word/search.html?q=empathy&submit.x=37&submit.y=29.

4. Brené Brown, *The Gifts of Imperfection: Let Go of Who You Think You're Supposed to Be and Embrace Who You Are* (Center City, MN: Hazelden), 19.

5. Eichenbaum and Orbach, *Between Women.*

6. Adrienne Harris, "Aggression, Envy, and Ambition: Circulating Tensions in Women's Psychic Life," *Gender and Psychoanalysis* 2 (1997): 291–325; Nancy

Chodorow, *The Reproduction of Mothering* (Berkeley and Los Angeles, CA: University of California Press, 1999).

7. Guy Winch, "7 Ways to Get Out of Guilt Trips," PsychologyToday.com (May 16, 2013), https://www.psychologytoday.com/blog/the-squeaky-wheel/201305/7-ways-get-out-guilt-trips; Guy Winch, *Emotional First Aid: Healing Rejection, Guilt, Failure, and Other Everyday Hurts* (New York: Plume, 2014).

8. Megan LeBoutillier, *No Is a Complete Sentence: Learning the Sacredness of Personal Boundaries* (New York: Ballantine Books, 1995).

9. Beatrice Beebe and Frank M. Lachmann, *The Origins of Attachment: Infant Research and Adult Treatment* (New York: Routledge, 2014); Judith Rustin, *Infant Research and Neuroscience at Work in Psychotherapy: Expanding the Clinical Repertoire* (New York: Norton, 2013).

11. WHY DO WOMEN FRIENDS HOLD GRUDGES *FOREVER?*: MANAGING ANGER, JUDGMENT, AND SHAME

1. Joyce F. Benenson and Richard W. Wrangham, "Cross-Cultural Sex Differences in Post-Conflict Affiliation Following Sports Matches," *Current Biology* 26 (2016): 2208–2212, doi:http://dx.doi.org/10.1016/j.cub.2016.06.024.

2. Cathi Hanauer, *The Bitch in the House: 26 Women Tell the Truth About Sex, Solitude, Work, Motherhood, and Marriage,* (New York: William Morris Paperbacks), 2003.

3. Jeanne Safer, "Broken Bridge: What Sparks the Demise of a Serious Friendship and What Can Be Salvaged from the Emotional Wreckage?" *Psychology Today* (March 1, 2016), 63.

4. Harriet Lerner, *Dance of Anger: A Woman's Guide to Changing the Patterns of Intimate Relationships,* (New York: HarperCollins, 2014).

5. N. Herrero, M. Gadea, G. Rodríguez-Alarcón, R. Espert, and A. Salvador, "What Happens When We Get Angry?: Hormonal, Cardiovascular, and Symmetrical Brain Responses," *Journal of Hormonal Behavior* 57 (2010): 276–283, doi:10.1016/j.yhbeh.2009.12.008.

6. Lerner. *The Dance of Anger* (New York: HarperCollins, 2014).

7. Douglas Stone, Bruce Patton, and Sheila Heen, *Difficult Conversations: How to Discuss What Matters Most* (New York: Penguin Books, 2010).

8. Sue Grafton, *X* (New York: G. P. Putnam's Sons, 2015).

9. Nancy Colier, "Why We Hold Grudges, and How to Let Them Go" PsychologyToday.com (2016), https://www.psychologytoday.com/blog/inviting-monkey-tea/201503/why-we-hold-grudges-and-how-let-them-go.

10. Gail Caldwell, *Let's Take the Long Way Home: A Memoir of Friendship* (New York: Random House, 2010), 27.

12. A HOLE IN YOUR HEART: DEALING
WITH ENDINGS AND LOSSES

1. Caldwell, *Let's Take the Long Way Home,* 201.
2. Ibid., 3.
3. American Psychological Association Help Center, "Grief: Coping with the Loss of Your Loved One" (2017), http://www.apa.org/helpcenter/grief.aspx
4. Ghislaine Boulanger, *Wounded by Reality: Understanding and Treating Adult-Onset Trauma* (New York: Mahwah, NJ), 2007.
5. John H. Harvey, Melanie K. Barnes, Heather R. Carlson, and Jeffrey Haig, "Held Captive by Their Memories: Managing Grief in Relationships," *Confronting Relationship Challenges,* Steve Duck (Ed.) (Thousand Oaks, CA: Sage Publications, 1995), 211–233.
6. Jacqueline P. Wiseman and Steve Duck, "Having and Managing Enemies," *Confronting Relationship Challenges,* Steve Duck (Ed.) (Thousand Oaks, CA: Sage Publications, 1995), 43–72.
7. Molly Castelloe, "A Holding Environment and Beyond 9/11," Psychology-Today.com (2010), https://www.psychologytoday.com/blog/the-me-in-we/201009/holding-environment-beyond-911.
8. Elisabeth Kübler-Ross, *On Death and Dying,* (New York: Scribner Classics, 1997); Vaughan Bell, "We All Grieve in Our Own Way," *The Guardian,* Saturday, November 24, 2012, https://www.theguardian.com/science/2012/nov/25/grief-mourning-psychology-customs.
9. Elisha Goldstein, *Uncovering Happiness: Overcoming Depression with Mindfulness and Self-Compassion* (New York: Atria Books, 2015).
10. NoViolet Bulawayo, *We Need New Names* (New York: Little, Brown, 2013), 212.
11. American Psychological Association Help Center, "Grief: Coping with the Loss of Your Loved One."
12. F. Diane Barth, "Listening to Words, Hearing Feelings: Links Between Eating Disorders and Alexithymia," *Clinical Social Work Journal* (2016): 38–50.
13. Jeanne Safer, *The Golden Condom: And Other Essays on Love Lost and Found* (New York: Picador, 2016). In her powerful novel *Before Everything* (New York: Viking, 2017) Victoria Redel movingly describes many different ways that this kind of unfolding and internalizing of complex, mixed emotions can occur over the course of a friend's illness and after her death.
14. Marilyn Peterson Haus, "For my friend, Michelle Gillett." Given at memorial service at the First Congregational Church, Stockbridge, Massachusetts, February 20, 2016.

13. THE SPECIAL JOY OF "FRIENDSHIP WISDOM"

1. H. S. Sullivan, *The Interpersonal Theory of Psychiatry* (New York: W.W. Norton, 1953).
2. Betsy Lerner, *The Bridge Ladies* (New York: HarperCollins, 2016), 170.
3. Ibid., 168.
4. Phil Garber, "Deep and Lasting Friendships Form in Jewish-Muslim Women's Group," *New Jersey Hills Observer-Tribune* (January 24, 2017), http://www.newjerseyhills.com/observer-tribune/news/deep-friendships-form-in-jewish-muslim-women-s-group/article_d3f832e0-03b8-5ffc-ab52-b076f1685e53.html.
5. Robert Stolorow, *Trauma and Human Existence* (New York: Analytic Press, 2007).
6. Ellen Ruderman and Carol Tosone, eds., *Contemporary Clinical Practice: The Holding Environment Under Assault* (New York: Springer, 2013).
7. Bulawayo, *We Need New Names.*
8. Sarah H. Matthews, *Friendships Through the Life Course* (Thousand Oaks, CA: Sage Publications, 1986); Steve Duck, Lee West, and Linda K. Acitelli, "Sewing the Field: The Tapestry of Relationships in Life and Research," *Handbook of Personal Relationships,* 2nd ed., Steve Duck (Ed.) (Hoboken, NJ: John Wiley and Sons, 1997), 1–27.
9. Betty Friedan, *The Fountain of Age,* (New York: Touchstone Press, 1993).
10. Edison J. Trickett and Rebecca M. Buchanan, "The Role of Personal Relationships in Transitions: Contributions of an Ecological Perspective," *Handbook of Personal Relationships,* Steve Duck (Ed.), 575–593.
11. Rachel Naomi Remen, *Kitchen Table Wisdom: Stories That Heal* (New York: Riverhead Books, 1996).
12. Michelle Gillett, "Old Friends," *The Berkshire Eagle,* October 29, 1991.

Index